An Introduction to
Medical Manipulation

An Introduction to Medical Manipulation

John K. Paterson, MB, BS, MRCGP
*currently Vice-President and Hon. Secretary of the British
Association of Manipulative Medicine and member of the
Scientific Advisory Committee of the International Federation of
Manual Medicine*

and

Loic Burn, BA, MRCS, LRCP, DPhysMed
*currently President of the British Association of Manipulative
Medicine, Hon. Secretary of the Scientific Section of the British
League against Rheumatism and member of Council of the Back
Pain Association*

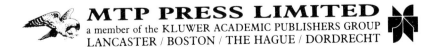

MTP PRESS LIMITED
a member of the KLUWER ACADEMIC PUBLISHERS GROUP
LANCASTER / BOSTON / THE HAGUE / DORDRECHT

Published in the UK and Europe by
MTP Press Limited
Falcon House
Lancaster, England

British Library Cataloguing in Publication Data

Paterson, John K.
  An introduction to medical manipulation.
  1. Manipulation (Therapeutics)
  I. Title II. Burn, Loic
  615.8′2   RM724

ISBN 0-85200-878-3

Published in the USA by
MTP Press
A division of Kluwer Boston Inc
190 Old Derby Street
Hingham, MA 02043, USA

Library of Congress Cataloging in Publication Data

Paterson, John K., 1921–
  An introduction to medical manipulation.

  Bibliography: p.
  Includes index.
  1. Manipulation (Therapeutics) I. Burn, Loic,
  1935–   . II. Title. [DNLM: 1. Joint Diseases—
  therapy. 2. Manipulation, Orthopedic. 3. Muscular
  Diseases—therapy. 4. Pain—therapy. 5. Spinal
  Diseases therapy. WE 725 P296i]
  RM724.P38 1985   615.8′2   85–137

ISBN 0-85200-878-3

Typeset and printed by Butler & Tanner Ltd, Frome and London.

Contents

Preface

We hope that this book will be of interest to all clinicians involved in the treatment of musculoskeletal problems, be they medical, paramedical or lay. It is primarily directed at general practitioners.

Musculoskeletal problems constitute the largest single group of conditions met with in general practice. There is at present a lack of teaching of the subject in Britain, in respect of both the nature of these ill-defined conditions and their therapy. With many years' experience of general practice, both of us are fully aware of the scale and importance of these issues. We seek to provide a wide and balanced review of the current state of knowledge in this field, culled from the available literature.

A method of clinical examination applicable to this group of conditions is presented. A collection of therapeutic manoeuvres suitable for use in general practice is described, with carefully worded texts, illustrated by photographs and diagrams, together with a variety of injection techniques, similarly illustrated. Drug therapy and other forms of treatment are discussed. We include sections on prophylaxis, together with further topics of relevance to general practice.

If the book appears overcritical of some ideas discussed, this is not our intention, but is rather the result of our understanding of the available literature. If we have omitted any relevant evidence, or if our reasoning is faulty, we will be happy to be so advised.

We would like to thank Mr Jim Norton, of the British League Against Rheumatism, and Group Captain Cedric Simons, of the Back Pain Association, for vetting that part of our material which pertains to those organizations.

Of the many colleagues who have lent help and advice, we wish in particular to thank Dr A. Maxwell Robertson and Professor Robert Maigne. However, our greatest debt of gratitude must be to Professor Barry Wyke, for his encouragement and painstaking criticism, and for doing us the honour of writing a foreword to this book.

14, Wimpole Street,   John K. Paterson
London W1M 7AB.   Loic Burn
September, 1984

Foreword

By Professor Barry Wyke, M.D.
Formerly Director of the Neurological Unit,
Royal College of Surgeons of England

Manipulative therapy is a technology based on the application of manual forces through bodily tissues with the object of relieving a variety of disorders, principally of the musculoskeletal system. It is one of the most ancient of therapies, having been practised (in some form or another) throughout human history; but in spite of this ancient lineage (or perhaps because of it), it has persisted as a largely empirical body of knowlege split into a variety of 'schools', each with its (sometimes fanatical) devotees.

This picture is now changing, however, as a result of the application of scientific investigation to the observations and procedures of manipulative therapy; and this book is a welcome British reflection of this change that should assist United Kingdom doctors in understanding the role of manipulative procedures in contemporary clinical practice. This is especially desirable, in that while countries such as Germany, France, Switzerland and The Netherlands each have a well-established medical speciality of Manual Medicine, such is not the case in Great Britain.

London,　　　　　　　　　　　　　　　　　　　　　Barry Wyke
January 1985

1
General Considerations

ORTHOPAEDIC NEUROLOGY I – HOW MANIPULATION WORKS

This presentation is based very largely on a series of lectures given by Professor B.D. Wyke in September 1983 in Zürich. In this, 20 years after the foundation of the specialty of articular neurology which encompasses the morphology, physiology, pathology and clinical features of joints, he gave a review of its current status.

By the time a patient feels pain, a very complex sequence of events has taken place. The gate theory, which has been established many years, was reviewed by Professor Wall in 1978 as follows.

'Information about the presence of injury is transmitted to the central nervous system by peripheral nerves. Certain small-diameter fibres will signal only on injury, while others with lower thresholds, increase their discharge frequency if the stimulus received reaches noxious levels.

'Cells of the spinal cord or fifth nucleus which are excited by these injury signals, are also facilitated or inhibited by other peripheral nerve fibres which carry information about innocuous events.

'Descending control systems originating in the brain modulate the excitability of the cells which transmit information about injury. Therefore the brain receives messages about injury by way of a gate control system which is influenced by: (1) injury signals, (2) other types of afferent impulse, and (3) descending control'[1].

The nerve endings in joints are internationally classified as Types 1-4. Types 1, 2 and 3 are corpuscular in type – that is they are nerve terminals enclosed in capsules with a variable number of layers. These are the mechano-receptors, converting mechanical forces applied to the nerve endings into nerve impulses, discharging into the central nervous system. Their response varies with the direction, velocity and amplitude of the forces applied to them, including those forces applied in therapeutic manipulation. Types 1 and 2 are embedded in the joint capsules and are, in fact, the only joint capsule mechanoceptors. Type 1 mechanoceptors are situated principally in the superficial layers, Type 2 deeper. Neither are in synovial tissues, there being no nerve endings in these tissues. Type 3 mechanoceptors are found only in ligaments; they are found in all ligaments.

The behaviour of any mechanoceptor, in whatever tissue it may be situated, is related to the thickness of its capsule. This determines the way in which it responds in terms of both time and resilience on movement, active or passive, to traction or to the application of external forces, such as manipulation. Adaptation is defined as the length of time for which a mechanoceptor will continue to discharge nerve impulses, when exposed to a mechanical force of constant intensity. Type 1 mechanoceptors are slowly adapting, Type 2 fast. Type 1 have thin capsules, Type 2 thicker, the general rule being that the thinner the capsule the more slowly will adaptation take place. A further significant difference between these two nerve endings is the way they behave, either at rest or when moved, actively or passively. Type 1 receptors fire constantly at rest, at about 15 Hz, whereas Type 2 do not fire at all at rest. Thus Type 1 receptors have a static discharge. However, the character of these discharges varies on movement according to the direction and amplitude of the forces applied to them. Thus Type 1 receptors have both static and dynamic discharges. Types 1 and 2 mechanoceptors have a feature in common, in that they have a low threshold, being very easily stimulated. Thus a force of approximately 3 grams is sufficient to stimulate a Type 1 mechanoceptor.

Since the tension in the joint capsules is greater than this, there is a static discharge from these particular mechanoceptors. Although Type 2 also have a low threshold, they have no static discharge; this is because their discharge is velocity dependent. That is to say, in order to recruit them, movements, active or passive, have to be rapid, and this is why they are known as acceleration mechanoceptors. The implication for the manipulator is obvious.

Type 3, the ligament mechanoceptors, have thin capsules – that is to say, they are slow adaptors. But they differ from Types 1 and 2 in that they have a high threshold. In order to induce them to discharge, forces of kilograms, not grams, have to be applied, and therefore they have no ·static discharge. They will only fire at the limits of range of movement, either active or passive, or on powerful traction or on forceful manipulation.

Type 4 nerve endings, the nociceptors, are those whose stimulation gives rise to the experience of pain. These are quite different from the mechanoceptors, in that they are non-capsulated. They are sub-divided into two types, Type 4a which are plexiform and found in the joint capsules and fat pads, and Type 4b which are free nerve endings found in ligaments. They are normally quiescent at rest or on movement. They are only fired on mechanical or chemical irri-tation, the former being very much more common, which is of inter-est to manipulators. The chemical substances which can stimulate these nerve endings include irritants such as prostaglandin-E, lactic acid, potassium ions, polypeptides and histamine. These substances appear in conditions of ischaemia and hypoxia, and also in inflam-matory exudates.

The afferent fibres transmitting nerve impulses generated via these various receptors enter the spinal cord, and it is now known that they divide into two rami, anterior and posterior. All nociceptor afferents are shunted to the anterior ramus, and all mechanoceptors to the posterior ramus. Nociceptive afferents give off many branches, but all give off one collateral branch which runs to the basal spinal nucleus. It is the axons of these nuclei that transmit nociceptive impulses on, up into the brain, and this is therefore the nociceptive gateway to the brain. For pain to be perceived, this barrier must be traversed. Whether this happens, and to what degree it happens, is dependent upon a peripheral modulating influence provided by the mechanoceptors. This input is derived mostly from muscle spindle, skin and joint mechanoceptors.

All mechanoceptor afferents give off a collateral branch to synapse with the apical nuclei. The axons from these nuclei then run for-ward to establish presynaptic relations with the terminals of the no-ciceptive afferents. A crucial factor is that the synaptic transmitter released from these apical spinal neurons onto the nociceptive presynaptic terminals is an endorphin which happens to be an in-hibitor. Therefore, nociceptive traversal of this barrier is inversely proportional to the incoming volume of mechanoceptor traffic. The greater this volume, the less, if any, pain is experienced. A further remarkable fact is that there is no local enzyme capable of breaking down this endorphin. Therefore it can only be washed away in the bloodstream, and it so happens that the blood supply in this area is the poorest in the central nervous system.

A number of treatments make use of this system of stimulating mechanoceptor input. The most ancient is massage. A second is the vibrator, the principle being to stimulate receptors in tissues from skin to periosteum. Because mechanoceptors are more sensitive than nociceptors, it is possible to stimulate the former and not the latter, the relevant level for most people being between 120 and 140 Hz. Another treatment which involves the same principle is transcutaneous nerve stimulation. In this instance it is the nerve trunks that are stimulated, rather than the receptors, but the principle is the same as with the vibrator; that is, to choose a frequency at which the more sensitive, larger fibres which contain the mechanoceptor afferents are stimulated, in preference to the smaller, more resistant nociceptive fibres. This proves very useful to the physician. Because of the endorphin and blood supply problem mentioned above, 20–30 minutes of stimulation frequently produces relief from pain for between 4 and 6 hours, or sometimes longer.

It seems clear that manipulation operates the same mechanism. Passive movements applied to the spine stimulate joint capsule mechanoceptors and muscle spindle receptors in the neighbourhood of the joints moved. It would seem from this that manipulation is probably as effective as massage, and that clinically it is far quicker to apply.

It should be observed that most osteopaths employ much articulation and other techniques which are, in fact, forms of gentle mobilization and massage, and many of them pride themselves on using no thrust or manipulative force at all. It also follows that, if this provides an explanation as to how manipulation works, the use, as many lay osteopaths claim, of many hundreds of techniques is unnecessary. The generation of a healthy mechanoceptor input is quite possible to achieve with relatively simple and few techniques, and these should be both easy to teach and widely applicable to general practice.

ORTHOPAEDIC NEUROLOGY 2 – A REVIEW OF CURRENT IDEAS RELATING TO MANIPULATION

To its adherents, osteopathy is a system of healing whose principal theme is that mechanical and structural abnormalities adversely affect the harmony and efficiency of the body. When the spine is manipulated, the principal concern is to remove any mechanical hindrance to the restoration of normal movements in the affected joints. This is because an imperfectly functioning structure predisposes to disease. 'Imperfect function in joints matters most in the spinal column because of the proximity of the spinal cord and spinal nerves. If these vital structures are adversely affected by faulty mechanics, then health is impaired and disease may ensue'[2].

The effects of intermittent compression and traction on nerves are particularly important to the osteopathic concept. The resultant centripetal effects of increased afferent discharge to the spinal cord contribute to the 'facilitated segment' at the same level. Centrifugal effects of autonomic stimulation lead to changes in the vasomotor, visceromotor and pseudomotor tone. 'The increased centrally summated state creates what is called a facilitated segment because the threshold for the efferent discharge is lowered and the transmission of impulses is therefore facilitated. These discharges lead to abnormal function, in the first place to hyperfunction, and later to hypofunction and then, if the abnormal stimuli persist for long enough, pathological changes can then ensue. The irritated spinal segment is vulnerable to other noxious influences and, even if a mechanical cause in itself is not sufficient to evoke abnormal responses, the combination of it with other factors is sufficient to produce abnormal symptoms. Mechanical lesions are aetiological in many diseases because adhesions weaken those viscera which are reflexly and segmentally linked with them. They cannot or should not be discounted in any disease[2].

'So we can contend that, by restoring normal mechanics, we are achieving in a natural way the restoration of autonomic balance by calming the stimulated and over-excitable segment'[2]. Thus manipulation is seen by the osteopaths to be more than a means, among others, of relieving mechanical pain in certain circumstances. A local vertebral abnormality can be detected, it can be treated by local methods and normal function restored. Under these circumstances related spinal cord segments are restored to normality, and it is claimed that potentially serious disease processes are averted or ameliorated. Another longstanding concept is that of autonomic pain – that is to say, pain that is experienced wholly through the autonomic system. All these concepts are a matter of faith, and it is interesting to see what light is thrown upon them by the work that has been carried out in recent years.

The first to consider is the concept of autonomic pain. Wyke showed, in 1970, that irritation of spinal joint nociceptors simultaneously evoked a large number of reflex alterations, including paravertebral muscle spasm and alterations in cardiovascular, respiratory and endocrine function[3]. That is to say that pain invariably involves both soma and viscera, and therefore the idea that autonomic pain can exist as a separate entity is not tenable. It has also been shown that any afferent fibre entering the spinal cord immediately divides into ascending and descending collateral branches extending for varying distances, sometimes the whole neuraxis, at whatever level the input reaches the cord. Further, given the complexity revealed in the gate theory, it is obvious that the extent to which this takes place in any given circumstance is wholly unpredictable. These ascending and descending branches form the propriospinal tracts and give off collateral branches to the spinal grey matter, to synapse with neurons in motorneuron pools or, more frequently, interneurons. Therefore all activity is instantly and unpredictably plurisegmental. The consequence of this to osteopathic theory is self-evident. There is, quite simply, no such thing as the facilitated cord segment.

Much is made in osteopathic literature of the significance of viscerosomatic and somaticovisceral reflexes, since these clearly imply a neurological involvement of visceral status. These are also assumed to be predominantly spinal. These reflexes, though they do exist, are very much more complex than this would suggest and involve, for example, hormonal changes. Moreover, there is now ample evidence that many of these changes take place in and are modified by the anterior and posterior nuclei of the hypothalamus. These reflexes are not predominantly spinal at all[4]. If neurology is seen to be plurisegmental, and these reflexes are shown to be not primarily spinal, it is difficult to see how a local lesion at a spinal segmental level, followed by local treatment, can have much – if any – influence on them. The significance for the medical manipulator is considerable. Up till now, there has been presented no evidence to counter the osteopathic explanations aimed at proving that manipulation affects the state of health in general. These arguments having been shown to be unrealistic, the status of manipulation must be seen in a new light. Thus it cannot, on existing evidence, be shown to be a system of healing, but it is simply a method of treatment for pain of mechanical origin.

SPINAL MOBILITY AND ITS RELEVANCE TO MANIPULATION

For the chiropractor, 'the first characteristic of the manipulatable lesion is restricted joint motion. This is the so-called fixation or blockage. The diagnosis of restricted joint motion is through palpation of movement between vertebrae or by motion X-ray. For example, the palpation of flexion–extension motion can be achieved by placing the fingers between the spinous processes and having the patient flex and extend the spine'[5]. The chiropractor seeks to find by palpation tissue changes, and in particular changes in mobility, at the segmental level assumed to be at fault.

For the osteopath, the keystone of his practice is the osteopathic spinal lesion, which is a condition of impaired mobility in an intervertebral joint. To quote Colin Dove, at the Colt Symposium of 1982, 'what the osteopath aims to do is to restore the normal functions of tissues, particularly movement where it is perceived to be lacking. Even if his assessment leads him to assume that the symptoms are arising at the level of hypermobility, he will seek to improve mobility elsewhere'[6]. This approach is entirely subjective. It is a matter of belief, and no evidence has ever been produced in support of this theory.

In the 1980 edition of *The Lumbar Spine and Back Pain* there is a chapter on sagittal mobility of the spine by Hilton. In his analysis of 103 postmortem specimens of the lower spine, he writes, 'At each disc level in both sexes there is a wide scatter of mobility values, but the mean mobility falls progressively from L5. However, the small fall shown by the mean is misleading, since the mobility in most individuals is to a varying degree irregularly distributed. Only 9 females and 7 males conformed to the mean mobility pattern, and of these 13 were aged less than 50 years.

'The irregularity in mobility pattern occurs irrespective of age and sex, and can be due to either reduction or increase in mobility at any level. These irregularities are often unpredictable from straight X-rays and do not necessarily reflect gross pathology, since they can occur in relatively healthy specimens'[7].

The objection that these findings might not be applicable in the living must be considered in the light of the fact that postmortem changes in mobility are likely to occur at much the same rate at all spinal levels. Hilton's work seems to indicate that variations in segmental mobility are exceedingly common and therefore will be found in similar proportions in back pain sufferers and among members of the community who are pain-free. Moll and Wright[8] observed spinal mobility *in vivo*. They found in normal subjects that there was a marked decrease in spinal mobility with age, and also a sex difference. They further found that the scatter not only varied between decades, but in each age group was considerable. The wide range of normal mobility was observed in flexion, extension and side-bending. This seems to confirm *in vivo* the findings of Hilton in the cadaver. If this is so, it follows that to use the detection of such variations as the basis of a comprehensive system of diagnosis and assessment of treatment is not legitimate. It seems to be a further demonstration of Troup's axiom that no sign, either clinical or radiological, that has been found in the back pain sufferer has not subsequently been demonstrated in pain-free members of the community.

INCIDENCE AND AETIOLOGY OF LOW BACK PAIN IN GENERAL TERMS

Anderson, in 1976, wrote that 'the range of labels used in connection with back pain is a fair reflection of medical ignorance and factional interest. Furthermore, it is virtually impossible to classify statistical data on sickness absence in a meaningful way ... specific surveys are difficult to compare in the absence of agreed semantics'[9]. In the light of this it is difficult to claim real statistical authority. Nevertheless, at the present time in the United Kingdom, almost 90 000 individuals registered as sick are away from work each day with back problems. This figure has reached its current level following a large increase over the past 5 years and is showing no sign at all of decreasing. The cost is around a billion pounds sterling a year in lost production, sickness benefits and medical treatment. One large-scale survey by Hay, in 1972, relating the incidence of low back pain to age, found that in both male and female the incidence increased radically between the ages of 20 and 40, thereafter remained static until the age of 60 and then declined[10]. Therefore the correlation between the incidence of back pain and age is not as clear cut as many suppose.

Several factors that have been found to be associated with increased absence from work due to back pain will be considered. They all increase the load on the spine, but, since they are often present at the same time, the association with any single factor is difficult to establish. With regard to heavy physical work and back pain, a study was carried out in Dundee comparing the incidence of these problems in nurses and teachers[11]. Although nursing is considered a heavier type of occupation than teaching, little difference was found between nurses and teachers in the overall prevalence of low back pain. However, low back pain presented earlier in nurses and it was largely precipitated by factors at work, whereas in teachers the incidence of back pain gradually increased with time, and it was generally non-occupational in origin. Several studies[12] indicate that heavy workloads have little effect on the incidence of low back pain, but have a much greater effect on the incidence of low back compensation and disability[13]. With regard to static work postures, several investigators have stressed the importance of prolonged sitting[14], driving vehicles[15], and also positions when the person is bending over his work[16]. It must be observed, however, that not all workers are in agreement. The association between low back pain and frequent bending and twisting is difficult to evaluate separately as lifting is usually also involved.

Troup, in 1970, found the combination mentioned above to be the most frequent cause of back injuries in England[17]. It is clearly established that back pain can be brought on by lifting, but the frequency of lifting incidents involved varies very considerably between studies[13]. Chaffin and Park, in 1973, found that workers involved in heavy manual lifting had about eight times the number of low back injuries compared with those with more sedentary work[18]. Many other research workers are in agreement. Any repetitive work increases, in general terms, the sickness absence rate[19], and low back pain also fits in with this axiom. This may explain, at least in part, why assembly line industries have a higher incidence of low back pain among their manual workers than among their office employees. With regard to vibration, there is evidence suggesting an increased risk of back pain in drivers of tractors[20], trucks[15] and buses, and in pilots[21]. Finally, psychological work factors involving monotony and work dissatisfaction have been found to increase the risk of back pain. Taylor, in 1968, observed that sickness absences increased in subjects with this problem, regardless of diagnosis[22].

Turning from occupational to individual factors in the aetiology of back pain, there are a number of issues to be considered. With regard to ageing, the work of Hay has already been mentioned[10]. The frequency of back pain symptoms appears to be maximal between the ages of 35 and 55[23], while sickness absence and symptom duration increase with increasing age. Sex factors seem to be without significance with respect to back pain with one exception. Women engaged in heavy physical work seem to be more prone to back pain than their male counterparts[24]. Recent work in Shropshire (Department of Spinal Disorders, 1982) shows that 'about 20% of females developed back pain in the first trimester with no previous history'[25]. Postural deformities such as scoliosis, kyphosis and leg length discrepancy do not seem to predispose to back pain[12,26]. On the other hand, subjects with scoliosis associated with apparent differences in leg length, who also have back pain, are commonly improved by the use of a heel raise, which suggests a correlation at least in a proportion of cases. Scoliosis has been particularly implicated by many people, but no hard evidence of a true association with back pain has so far been established[27]. With regard to height, tallness has been found to be associated with back pain in some studies[28]. Obesity, unless extreme, has not[29]. Farfan, in 1973, found there was no correlation between obesity and disc disease and degeneration[30]. With regard to muscular strength and physical fitness, results are variable, Nachemson and Lindt, in 1968, being notable in finding no correlation[27]. Cady, in 1979, concluded from a study of Los Angeles firemen that physical fitness had a significant preventative effect on the occurrence of back pain, but there were several other differences between the two groups of people he studied, complicating the interpretation of these findings[31]. Radiological and psychological factors are considered elsewhere. It is clear that, while much valuable information has been obtained which is of help in prophylaxis, individual and workplace factors are often difficult to isolate.

REFERRED PAIN, REFERRED TENDERNESS AND BACK PAIN SYNDROMES

As long ago as 1939, Kellgren demonstrated the existence of referred pain following the injection of hypertonic saline solutions into the vertebral connective tissues[32]. In 1951 Frykholm, in his operations on cervical spines under local anaesthesia, found on stimulating the dorsal root that the patient experienced pain in the distribution of the dermatome[33]. If the anterior motor root was stimulated, the patient felt a pain situated in muscles which had been painful and tender before operation. In 1959, Cloward described referral of pain to periscapular areas on injecting for discography under local anaesthesia into the anterior parts of various cervical discs C3/C4, C4/C5, C5/C6 and C6/C7[34]. He identified the painful areas as being C3/C4 for the upper fibres of the trapezius, C4/C5 the upper scapular medial border, C5/C6 the middle of the medial border of the scapula and C6/C7 medial at the inferior angle. These authors not only demonstrated the existence of referred pain, but fell into the error of assuming that the site of the referred pain gave a clear indication of the site of origin. This has been shown not to be the case – not only by Holt in 1964[35], but also by Klafta and Collis in 1969[36], who performed 549 cervical disc injections over a 10-year period, in an endeavour to evaluate the diagnostic usefulness of pain associated with discography. Pain similar to the presenting symptoms was produced in 22% of cases, dissimilar pain in 67% and no pain at all in 11% of cases. Kirk and Denny-Brown, in 1970[37], and subsequently Denny-Brown et al., in 1973[38], have shown experimentally that an isolated dermatome can vary enormously in extent and, indeed, that the dermatomes should be considered as a neurophysiological entity which can vary almost from moment to moment. Last, in 1978, wrote that 'the dermatome charts of the limb are probably as accurate today as maps of the world were in the 16th Century'[39]. Thus, Mooney and Robertson (1976), 'It is apparent to us that the localization of pain in the low back, buttock and leg is a non-specific finding'[40]. Discussing the apophyseal joint syndrome, they say 'on the other hand, the very same referral pattern can no doubt be caused by irritation within the spinal canal'[40]. Bourdillon (1973) wrote that 'a remarkable property of referred pain is that it can appear to be exactly the same when produced by either two (or

11

more) separate sources'[41]. When one considers the nociceptive innervation of lumbosacral tissues, for example, it is quite clear that any posture maintained over a prolonged period of time can affect muscles, fasciae, ligaments and articular capsules. All these nociceptor systems are capable, severally or together, of stimulating painful paravertebral muscle spasm.

Tenderness is very commonly associated with low back pain and referred pain. 'Referred pain may or may not be accompanied by secondary hyperaesthesiae'[42]. Macnab, in 1977, found that injection of hypertonic saline into the lumbosacral supraspinous ligament could not only radiate pain down the leg but could also be associated with tender points in varying sites commonly situated over the sacro-iliac joint and in the outer quadrant of the buttock[43].

O'Brien, in 1979, discovered that on palpating the lumbosacral promontory via the abdominal wall he found tenderness in more than three quarters of patients with low back pain. In a controlled group of 50 asymptomatic individuals, only two exhibited tenderness and both of them had experienced back pain in the preceding 3 months[44]. Frykholm[33] and Cloward[34] both demonstrated referred tenderness. Unfortunately, the diagnostic use of this phenomenon is as restricted as that of referred pain. 'The certain identification of minor paravertebral muscle strains by palpation is not as easy as might appear, since the phenomenon of referred tenderness can bedevil the most careful examination'[45].

Therefore it can be seen that to use the site of pain or tenderness as a means of arriving at a specific diagnosis, indicating a specific tissue, is unrealistic in most of the cases of back pain that we meet. Over the years many syndromes, i.e. collections of symptoms and signs, have been presented as being reliable diagnostic tools. Examples are sudden backache, impacted synovial meniscoid villus, the cocktail party syndrome, the locking of an arthrotic facet joint, the adolescent acute back and slow onset backache and sciatica, or the equinox syndrome. In view of the material presented, such syndromes must be regarded with very considerable doubt. Indeed, in this area it is doctors themselves who have, sadly, greatly contributed to the confusion which is so marked a feature of this field. 'The range of labels used in connection with back pain is a fair reflection of medical ignorance and of factional interests'[46]. Moreover, this has had the disadvantage, among others, of persuading the clinician that he has the correct diagnosis of the patient's problems and therefore, in his persisting in a particular line of treatment which, in view of the above evidence, is not reasonable. Given the existing state of knowledge, diagnostic as well as therapeutic empiricism should be the order of the day until more information becomes available.

TRIGGER POINTS

The existence of palpable and tender nodules in muscles has long been known. Froriep in 1843, in Weimar, published material relating to them and they have been a source of much study in Germany ever since[47]. In Britain they have been frequently described as 'fibrositis', firstly by Gowers in 1904[48]. Another significant paper was published by Copeman and Ackerman in 1947, in which it was proposed that they were due to herniations of lobulated fat[49]. Travell first published a paper in 1942 on the study of these trigger points, in patients with shoulder difficulties, and has published many papers since on this and allied subjects[50]. No one so far has been able to identify these problems histologically. It is therefore reasonable to suggest the term 'fibrositis' should not be used, since its existence has never been proven[51].

'One of the most poorly understood phenomena relating to chronic pain syndromes is the focal hyperirritability of tissues related to painful areas of the body. These areas are generally classed as trigger points and frequently represent areas of referred pain and autonomic nerve dysfunction'[52]. With regard to referred pain, while there is frequently a definite association, the site or sites to which pain or tenderness are referred are unpredictable. It is for this reason that referred pain and tenderness may be used only with reservation as diagnostic tools. 'Trigger points associated with myofascial and visceral pains often lie within the areas of referred pain but many are located at a distance from them'[53]. As long ago as 1938, Steindler and Luck studied 451 cases of low back pain with pain referred to the leg on localized palpation in the lumbosacral region[54]. In 228 of them, points were located where needling produced pain felt both locally and referred. Both types of pain were relieved by injection of local anaesthetic in the lumbosacral tender point. It is now generally accepted that the eradication of these points by injection or needling does not indicate that its source has been identified[43]. Nevertheless, such treatments are of considerable help. It has also been shown that injecting saline is about as effective as is injecting local anaesthetic and that simply using a dry needle is only slightly less effective than saline[55]. The possibility of a correlation with acupuncture has been studied, notably by Melzack in 1977, who wrote that 'a remarkably high degree (71%) of correspondence was found[53]. This close correlation suggests that trigger points and acupuncture points of pain, although discovered independently and named differently, represent the same phenomenon and can be explained in terms of the same underlying neuromechanisms'. Complexities of reference have been highlighted by Simons in 1975, who showed that a lower thoracic point may refer pain to the lower buttock while an upper lumbar point may refer pain to an area over the upper buttock[55]. In 1976, Maigne demonstrated that upper cervical problems could not only cause frontal headache but also referred tenderness to eyebrow tissues and that both symptoms and signs could be eradicated by treatment to the upper cervical spine[56]. It is well worth while seeking these points, since they are common, and treatment of them is simple, harmless and frequently of great benefit to the patient.

SOME PSYCHOLOGICAL ASPECTS OF VERTEBRAL PAIN

The close connection between psychological problems and pain can be seen when one comes to consider the definition of pain. This is defined by Wood as 'an emotional response to an afferent input'[51]. The relationship between emotion and pain was clearly observed by Montaigne in 1580, when he wrote that 'Nous sentons plus un coup de rasoir du chirurgien que dix coups d'épée en la chaleur du combat.' ('We feel a cut from a barber's razor more keenly than ten sword wounds received in the heat of battle.') A more extensive definition of pain is 'an unpleasant sensory and emotional experience associated with actual or potential tissue damage or described in terms of such damage'[57]. This emphasizes that pain is always given a location, however imprecise, by the patient. In the seventeenth century, the philosopher Spinoza defined pain as a 'localized form of sorrow'.

The incidence of pain in psychiatric practice is higher than one might imagine. Almost two thirds of psychiatric patients complain of pain or suffer from it either as a minor or major problem[58]. If one considers those patients who have chronic pain as a major complaint, a probable psychiatric illness and no physical lesion to account for their pain, about 30% will have prominent hysterical characteristics. 'Some people will have a symptom, including headache or sickness or other pain because of an unconscious motive. That is the idea I am working on when I say that some patients have pain on an hysterical basis'[58]. A quarter will have major anxiety symptoms or syndromes, and 10–15% will have depression[59,60]. Sternbach used the Minnesota Multiphasic Personality Inventory (MMPI), which is the best-established psychological test used to measure personality in the USA in chronic pain sufferers. This showed that, using measures of hypochondriacal behaviour, there was great similarity between the pattern of the hysterical patient and the back pain patient[61]. That is, that the patient was quite disturbed, and that his attention was devoted to the body. Following treatment, either medical or surgical, the scores tended to drop and the abnormalities decline. The longer the history of pain, the greater the abnormalities detected. This tells us nothing about aetiology but, to quote Merskey, 'Psychiatric patients with no physical lesions can have a lot of pain and we can see that personality factors and other aspects of neurotic illness are common in producing pain'[62].

In an investigation on patients who had definite physical lesions as a cause of their pain, such as post-herpetic neuralgia etc, and in others who had chronic pain but no recognizable physical signs, Merskey found that patients who had demonstrable physical abnormalities scored higher on scales of neuroses than patients who were only neurotic. This indicates that psychological disturbances can be secondary to pain. This was reinforced in going into the psychological background of the people involved, because it was found that those who had purely neurotic problems were more likely to have, for example, disturbed childhoods, than those who had psychological problems clearly secondary to their physical troubles[63]. In a profile of the kind of patients he expected to see who had pain and associated psychiatric phenomena, he found that schizophrenia was hardly ever associated. In the severely chronic group, patients had hysterical symptoms or personality traits, a great concern about their bodies and a poor response to treatment, psychological or physical. This group tended to do badly if subjected to surgery.

15

Discussing this work, Professor Merskey writes of patients with pain 'who do not have any recognizable (physical) lesion'.

In the past, numerous patients have been dismissed as not exhibiting abnormal physical signs as a direct result of those signs having been unsought due to their being unknown. In manipulative practice, it is common, for example, to see patients with headache of vertebral origin who have been labelled neurotic, who do in fact exhibit the palpatory signs of Maigne. It seems to us that a proportion of patients in such studies as we have quoted assumed to have pain of wholly psychological origin might well have exhibited positive physical signs on local examination.

In summary, the above material relates to chronic pain sufferers and therefore may not be wholly relevant to the kind of episodic problems mainly met with in general practice. Nevertheless, psychological problems and pain are clearly closely interrelated, and it is often difficult to decide which is primary and which secondary. The latter group is particularly important. Because of it, one should be very reluctant to assume, in a patient who does not respond to physical treatment readily, and who has evidence of psychological abnormalities, that the problem is wholly psychological and not physical. This is commonly done at present.

INDICATIONS, CONTRAINDICATIONS AND DANGERS

Indications

Symptoms

Because of the phenomenon of referred pain, vertebral problems can project symptoms over a disconcertingly wide area. Spinal problems in the neck commonly cause pain in the head, face, neck, upper trunk and arms. The thoracic spine can refer to the buttock and the lumbar spine to the leg, hip and perineum. See further material in Chapter 3, Thoracic Symptomatology Section, and Chapter 4, Classification of Low Back Pain section.

T6 can cause epigastric pain; T7 pain in the gall bladder area; T8 the kidneys; T10 and T11 ureter and bladder pain.

Thus visceral disease can be simulated, and errors of diagnosis and sometimes major surgery may follow. This is probably because, outside the specialities of rheumatology and orthopaedic surgery, the state of training with regard to musculoskeletal and vertebral problems is, sadly, surprisingly poor. It also explains the confusion that exists concerning the relationship between the spine and organic disease, which could to an extent be avoided if the former were more frequently, and particularly locally, examined.

See Chapter 3, Thoracic Symptomatology section, and Chapter 4, Classification of Low Back Pain Section.

Signs

Global movement
These are flexion, extension, rotation, lateral flexion. A free and symmetrical range by no means excludes spinal problem.

Palpatory tests
These are used to detect local tissue, ligament and muscle induration and tenderness. Pressure tests over the spinous processes and apophyseal joints seek local tenderness. These tests can indicate the site of a 'painful segmental disorder'. This term is deliberately vague, as further precision of diagnosis is usually impossible in our present state of knowledge.

Indication for manipulation
The demonstration and localization of a 'painful segmental disorder' is the indication for manipulation.

Contraindications

In view of the simplistic nature of the indications, the contraindications are most important and can be subdivided into two categories: (1) clinical and (2) technical.

Clinical
Fracture, neoplasm, infection, inflammatory disease and vascular problems are all absolute contraindications. Therefore, a careful diagnosis must be made, if need be with appropriate radiological or laboratory investigations. Secondaries may be derived from breast, lung, kidney, prostate and thyroid. When inflammatory diseases are active, manipulation is useless, painful and possibly dangerous. To

spend time manipulating active Scheuermann's disease or ankylosing spondylitis is to deny appropriate treatment, which is quite different. Nowhere is this more dramatically illustrated than with polymyalgia rheumatica, where to withhold the correct treatment is to risk retinal artery thrombosis and thereby blindness. Thus fracture and major pathology must be excluded.

There are several specific exclusions.

(1) The rheumatoid neck must never be manipulated, as life could be at risk, by the posterior dislocation of the odontoid process through a weakened or ruptured transverse ligament.

(2) The history is particularly important in eliminating neurological or vascular conditions. Thus 'drop attacks' and vertigo are highly significant. The principal danger is basilar artery thrombosis. In this situation a careful history is of paramount importance, as the so-called postural tests of hyperextension and full rotation have been known to cause major neurological accidents (Wyke, B.D., personal communication, 1984). Therefore, it is on history alone that these conditions should be suspected. It has recently been shown that 70% of these conditions are not due to arterial disease but in fact to proprioceptive distortions in the cervical spine[64]. Nevertheless, unless an arteriogram is performed and shown to be negative, because of the dangers, manipulation must be withheld in all such cases.

(3) *Grisel's syndrome*[65]. It has been demonstrated radiologically, notably by Gutmann in 1970[66], that in children with upper respiratory tract infections this syndrome can frequently involve hypermobility of the upper cervical spine. Therefore, in such cases, manipulation is strongly contraindicated.

(4) Cervical myelopathy must be borne in mind. The vascular supply to the spinal cord is only just adequate. Therefore, a spinal cord already ischaemic should not have manipulative techniques inflicted upon it.

(5) The same exclusion applies to thoracic myelopathy.

(6) With regard to the lumbar spine, a careful history and examination must be taken to exclude sphincter problems and saddle

anaesthesia, both absolute contraindications to manipulation, and indeed indications for *immediate* surgical referral.

Technical
Here there is no question of absolute contraindication. The decision is one of choosing the appropriate technique or of abstaining.

Dangers of manipulation

We have come across one recent case of near disaster in the neck. The patient was being treated by an osteopath, suffered brainstem damage and subsequently recovered[67].

We have been unable to find more than one instance of damage caused by manipulation of the thoracic or lumbar spine. This was reported by Jennett[68], and was a case of sphincter disturbance following lumbar manipulation under general anaesthesia.

In the 1982 edition of Cyriax's *Textbook of Orthopaedic Medicine* there are references to 21 reports of injury associated with vertebral manipulation. Of these, 14 refer specifically to chiropractic manipulation, the remaining seven being of unspecified nature[69-89].

As there are in excess of 25 000 chiropractors in the USA alone, the incidence of disaster is minute[90]. However, it is doubtful if any of these clinicians was aware of the pre-existing vascular pathology.

Despite the extremely low reported incidence of brainstem and spinal cord damage related to manipulation, the potential damage is so serious as to make the teaching of the contraindications to manipulation of the first importance. This applies equally to medical, paramedical and lay manipulators.

In this context, it is worth emphasizing the importance of taking an adequate history, and that postural testing of the cervical spine must be eschewed (Wyke, B.D., personal communication, 1984).

CLINICAL HISTORY AND DATA RECORDING

Those involved in the practice of medical manipulation grow accustomed to doing things very much their own way, evolving their own particular techniques in relation to their own physical and emotional make-up and in relation to the physical limitations of the environment within which they work. Tall clinicians may prefer sitting techniques, those with cramped consulting accommodation may be unable to get to the end of the couch. They must also modify techniques to suit individual patients. To some extent this is inevitable but, when this individuality spills over into history taking and data recording, two important results follow. First, without the advantage of a disciplined framework within which to record relevant data, the risk of failing to ask pertinent questions or to make observations is increased. Second, in the absence of a uniform system of data recording, comparison of data from different observers is rendered unnecessarily difficult, if not impossible.

It is clearly necessary to learn, accept and practise an overall methodology embracing history taking, examination and data recording, designed to minimize the risk of missing factors relevant to making therapeutic decisions. An adequate history must afford the doctor a picture of the patient encompassing far more than gender, age group, occupation and mode of onset and course of symptoms. In a group of conditions much affected by posture, it is necessary to have a clear view of the overall habit and mode of life. To this end clinical history and examination data sheets are presented on pages 22–31.

Routine administrative data in respect of patient and doctor must be written in full. This involves 20 items for the computer. Habit, at work and at home, in relation to driving motor cars and sporting activities, involves a further 23 items, requiring very little writing and a few ticks (most likely between five and ten.) Most of this may be elicited and entered by ancillary staff, if desired.

Previous related episodes require a date for the first attack, a few words of description, a maximum of five ticks and a figure for segmental level (as a topographical labelling device only), in up to three boxes. Similarly, non-related history is entered mainly by ticks. The whole of previous therapy is entered by ticks, providing a tabulated review of both treatments given and results obtained, together with the category of therapist.

The initial history of the present episode is dealt with by a few ticks and a few words. Regarding pain and altered sensation, provision is made for assessment prior to therapy and after, and also for assessment at up to four follow-up consultations. Current therapy to the time of initial consultation is entered largely by ticking the appropriate boxes, only side-effects requiring the use of words, apart from identification of the drug. Provision is made for comments.

Finally, the first sheet commences data recording of physical findings in respect of posture and apparent leg length inequality, again largely by means of a few ticks.

Except for identification of the patient, cervical and lumbar movements are the first to be entered on the second sheet, and, as with the history of the present episode, provision is made for assessment initially and after the first treatment, as well as at up to four follow-up appointments.

The same provision is made for assessment in the sections recording skin drag, loss of power, tendon reflexes (and plantars), skin rolling and increased muscle tone. This is also the case for supraspinous ligament tenderness, pain provoked by transverse pressure on the spinous processes and deep zygoapophyseal joint tenderness.

In use, these data sheets will be found to require entries on average in less than 10% of the boxes, of which entries roughly 25% will be written in words, maybe most of these by ancillary staff, the remainder in either ticks or figures.

Recorded in this way, the overall time for writing notes is substantially reduced; coupled with an increased volume of data recorded, a continuity of observation is provided at follow-up and all data are readily programmable for computer storage and recall, either as a means of keeping clinical records or as a preliminary to research.

It is hoped that the complexity of this form of data recording will be reduced following the identification of irrelevant data by means of a pilot study.

KFC Data Sheet I

PATIENTS NAME 01

ADDRESS 02

.... 03

.... 04

TELEPHONE 05

DOCTOR'S NAME 06

ADDRESS 07

.... 08

.... 09

TELEPHONE 10

Date first seen

| 11 |
| 12 |

Date of birth

Male [13]   Female [14]

Serial No. [15]

Dominant hand L [16]   R [17]

Peculiar Features

| 18 |
| 19 |
| 20 |

HABIT

Work [21]			
Heavy	Awkward	Light	Sitting +	SE
22	23	24	25	26

Home			
Slave	Shopping +	Garden +	Under 5's
27	28	29	30

Car [31]					
Short	Long	Auto	P/St	0 – 5000	5 – 15000	15 – 25000	More
32	33	34	35	36	37	38	39

	40

Sports	
41	42
	43

PREVIOUS RELATED EPISODES

First attack [44]				45	
Sudden	C	T	L	Bed	Restricted	Off work	Recurring	Worsening	Improving
46	47	48	49	50	51	52	53	54	55
									56

NON-RELATED HISTORY

Labours		Infants		
Normal	57	Largest	59	Kg
Abnormal	58	Smallest	60	Kg

Operations (with year)		
61		62
63		64

Injuries involving fracture	L	R
Cranial	65	66
Vertebro-pelvic	67	68
Brachial	69	70
Crural	71	72

Soft-tissue injuries	L	R
Cranial	73	74
Vertebro-pelvic	75	76
Brachial	77	78
Crural	79	80

MEDICAL CONDITIONS

	Past	Current
Malignant disease	81	82
Psoriasis	83	84
Gout	85	86
Diabetes mellitus	87	88
Steroid therapy	89	90
Rheumatoid arthritis	91	92
Ankylosing spondylitis	93	94
Sero-negative arthropathy	95	96

	Past	Current
Osteo-arthrosis	97	98
Osteo-porosis	99	100
Osteo-malacia	101	102
Osteo-chondritis	103	104
Polymyalgia rheumatica	105	106
Vascular disease	107	108
Anti-coagulant therapy	109	110
	111	112

PREVIOUS THERAPY

PREVIOUS THERAPY	Improved	ISQ	Worse	Doctor	Physio	Osteo	Other
Heat + exercises	113	114	115	116	117	118	119
SWD, U/S or I/F	120	121	122	123	124	125	126
Manipulation: painful	127	128	129	130	131	132	133
Manipulation: painless	134	135	136	137	138	139	140
Manipulation: under GA	141	142	143	144	145	146	147
Collar, corset etc	148	149	150	151	152	153	154
Traction: sustained	155	156	157	158	159	160	161
Traction: intermittent	162	163	164	165	166	167	168
Traction: continuous	169	170	171	172	173	174	175
Injections	176	177	178	179	180	181	182
Surgery	183	184	185	186	187	188	189
Other	190	191	192	193	194	195	196
	197	198	199	200	201	202	203

PRESENT EPISODE

Sudden onset	204
Duration, days	205
Duration, weeks	206
Duration, months	207
Duration, years	208

Unexplained weight loss	209
Drop attacks	210
Vertigo	211
Saddle anaesthesia	212
Sphincter problems	213

Precipitating factors	
	214
	215
	216
	217

PAIN

| Severity | | | | Level | Initial | | | | | | After therapy | | | | | | | | | | | |
+	++	+++	++++		L	M	R	L	M	R	L	M	R	L	M	R	L	M	R	L	M	R
218	219	220	221	Cranial	222	223	224	225	226	227	288	289	290	309	310	311	330	331	332	351	352	353
228	229	230	231	Cervical	232	233	234	235	236	237	291	292	293	312	313	314	333	334	335	354	355	356
238	239	240	241	Brachial	242	243	244	245	246	247	294	295	296	315	316	317	336	337	338	357	358	359
248	249	250	251	Thoracic	252	253	254	255	256	257	297	298	299	318	319	320	339	340	341	360	361	362
258	259	260	261	Lumbar	262	263	264	265	266	267	300	301	302	321	322	323	342	343	344	363	364	365
268	269	270	271	Sacral	272	273	274	275	276	277	303	304	305	324	325	326	345	346	347	366	367	368
278	279	280	281	Crural	282	283	284	285	286	287	306	307	308	327	328	329	348	349	350	369	370	371

ALTERED SENSATION

| Level | Initial | | | | | | After therapy | | | | | | | | | | | |
	L	M	R	L	M	R	L	M	R	L	M	R	L	M	R	L	M	R
Cranial	372	373	374	375	376	377	414	415	416	435	436	437	456	457	458	477	478	479
Cervical	378	379	380	381	382	383	417	418	419	438	439	440	459	460	461	480	481	482
Brachial	384	385	386	387	388	389	420	421	422	441	442	443	462	463	464	483	484	485
Thoracic	390	391	392	393	394	395	423	424	425	444	445	446	465	466	467	486	487	488
Lumbar	396	397	398	399	400	401	426	427	428	447	448	449	468	469	470	489	490	491
Sacral	402	403	404	405	406	407	429	430	431	450	451	452	471	472	473	492	493	494
Crural	408	409	410	411	412	413	432	433	434	453	454	455	474	475	476	495	496	497

CURRENT THERAPY

Preparation	Dose	Frequency	Result			Side effects
			Good	Moderate	Poor	
498	499	500	501	502	503	504
505	506	507	508	509	510	511
512	513	514	515	516	517	518
519	520	521	522	523	524	525

COMMENTS

526
527
528

EXAMINATION   Posture

	AP			Lateral		
	C	T	L		C	T	L
Erect	529	530	531	Erect	544	545	546
Side bend L	532	533	534	Flexed	547	548	549
Side bend R	535	536	537	Extended	550	551	552
Rotation L	538	539	540	Protracted	553	554	555
Rotation R	541	542	543	Retracted	556	557	558

APPARENT LEG LENGTH INEQUALITY

	Initial		After therapy	
	L	R	L	R
Less than 1cm	559	560	567	568
1 – 2cm	561	562	569	570
2 – 3cm	563	564	571	572
More than 3cm	565	566	573	574

KFC Data Sheet II

PATIENT'S NAME 01

SERIAL NO. 02

CERVICAL MOVEMENTS

Movement	Degree	Before		After										
		L	R	L	R	L	R	L	R	L	R	L	R
Extension	Less than 30°	03		21		39		57		75		93	
	30° – 60°	04		22		40		58		76		94	
	More than 60°	05		23		41		59		77		95	
Flexion	Less than 30°	06		24		42		60		78		96	
	30° – 60°	07		25		43		61		79		97	
	More than 60°	08		26		44		62		80		98	
Side Bending	Less than 30°	09	10	27	28	45	46	63	64	81	82	99	100
	30° – 60°	11	12	29	30	47	48	65	66	83	84	101	102
	More than 60°	13	14	31	32	49	50	67	68	85	86	103	104
Rotation	Less than 30°	15	16	33	34	51	52	69	70	87	88	105	106
	30° – 60°	17	18	35	36	53	54	71	72	89	90	107	108
	More than 60°	19	20	37	38	55	56	73	74	91	92	109	110

LUMBAR MOVEMENTS

	Before		After		Degree								
	L	R	L	R		L	R	L	R	L	R	L	R
Extension	111		129		Less than 30°	147		165		183		201	
	112		130		30° – 60°	148		166		184		202	
	113		131		More than 60°	149		167		185		203	
Flexion	114		132		Less than 30°	150		168		186		204	
	115		133		30° – 60°	151		169		187		205	
	116		134		More than 60°	152		170		188		206	
Side Bending	117	118	135	136	Less than 30°	153	154	171	172	189	190	207	208
	119	120	137	138	30° – 60°	155	156	173	174	191	192	209	210
	121	122	139	140	More than 60°	157	158	175	176	193	194	211	212
Rotation	123	124	141	142	Less than 30°	159	160	177	178	195	196	213	214
	125	126	143	144	30° – 60°	161	162	179	180	197	198	215	216
	127	128	145	146	More than 60°	163	164	181	182	199	200	217	218

SKIN DRAG

	Before		After									
	L	R	L	R	L	R	L	R	L	R	L	R
Cervical	219	220	225	226	231	232	237	238	243	244	249	250
Thoracic	221	222	227	228	233	234	239	240	245	246	251	252
Lumbar	223	224	229	230	235	236	241	242	247	248	253	254

REDUCED POWER

	Before		After									
	L	R	L	R	L	R	L	R	L	R	L	R
Cervical	255	256	263	264	271	272	279	280	287	288	295	296
Thoracic	257	258	265	266	273	274	281	282	289	290	297	298
Lumbar	259	260	267	268	275	276	283	284	291	292	299	300
	261	262	269	270	277	278	285	286	293	294	301	302

SENSORY LOSS

	Before		After									
	L	R	L	R	L	R	L	R	L	R	L	R
Cervical	303	304	311	312	319	320	327	328	335	336	343	344
Thoracic	305	306	313	314	321	322	329	330	337	338	345	346
Lumbar	307	308	315	316	323	324	331	332	339	340	347	348
Sacral	309	310	317	318	325	326	333	334	341	342	349	350

TENDON REFLEXES

	Before		After									
	L	R	L	R	L	R	L	R	L	R	L	R
Biceps	351	352	361	362	371	372	381	382	391	392	401	402
Triceps	353	354	363	364	373	374	383	384	393	394	403	404
Knee	355	356	365	366	375	376	385	386	395	396	405	406
Ankle	357	358	367	368	377	378	387	388	397	398	407	408
Plantar	359	360	369	370	379	380	389	390	399	400	409	410

STRESS TEST OF SI LIGAMENTS

	Before		After									
	L	R	L	R	L	R	L	R	L	R	L	R
Ilio-lumbar	411	412	417	418	423	424	429	430	435	436	441	442
Sacro-Iliac	413	414	419	420	425	426	431	432	437	438	443	444
Sacro-Tuberous	415	416	421	422	427	428	433	434	439	440	445	446

SKIN ROLLING

	Before		After									
	L	R	L	R	L	R	L	R	L	R	L	R
Cervical	447	448	453	454	459	460	465	466	471	472	477	478
Thoracic	449	450	455	456	461	462	467	468	473	474	479	480
Lumbar	451	452	457	458	463	464	469	470	475	476	481	482

INCREASED MUSCLE TONE

	Before		After									
	L	R	L	R	L	R	L	R	L	R	L	R
Cervical	483	484	489	490	495	496	501	502	507	508	513	514
Thoracic	485	486	491	492	497	498	503	504	509	510	515	516
Lumbar	487	488	493	494	499	500	505	506	511	512	517	518

SPRINGING

Before	After				
519	521	523	525	527	529
520	522	524	526	528	530

SUPRASPINOUS LIGAMENT TENDERNESS

	Before	After				
Thoracic	531	533	535	537	539	541
Lumbar	532	534	536	538	540	542

LATERAL SPINOUS PROCESS PRESSURE

	Before		After									
	L	R	L	R	L	R	L	R	L	R	L	R
Thoracic	543	544	547	548	551	552	555	556	559	560	563	564
Lumbar	545	546	549	550	553	554	557	558	561	562	565	566

APOPHYSEAL JOINT TENDERNESS

	Before		After									
	L	R	L	R	L	R	L	R	L	R	L	R
Cervical	567	568	573	574	579	580	585	586	591	592	597	598
Thoracic	569	570	575	576	581	582	587	588	593	594	599	600
Lumbar	571	572	577	578	583	584	589	590	595	596	601	602

THERAPY

	Initial				
Manipulation	603	608	613	618	623
Injection – Various	604	609	614	619	624
Injection – Epidural	605	610	615	620	625
Traction	606	611	616	621	626
Other	607	612	617	622	627

LOCAL EXAMINATION

The initial examination of the spine is based on the routine, orthodox, rheumatological and orthopaedic methods which are outlined
in the regional sections of this book. Our method, like Maigne's, is
essentially a system of local examination of the spine. It is derived
very largely from that originally devised by Professor Maigne. We
are very grateful to him for having discussed the matter with us,
although he differs from us on certain issues. While he lays emphasis
on referral of pain and tenderness within the myotome, sclerotome
and dermatome of the relevant nerve root, we believe these phenomena to be more widespread.

The principal instance of localization being of importance is when
a disc may require surgery, and then the methods are neurological
and radiological, rather than palpatory. Recent work demonstrates
this to be very much less common than previously believed. One
looks for a site of 'painful segmental disorder'. Its nature is a matter
for hypothesis and conjecture. What are looked for are local signs
of abnormal function, with two objects – first, to determine the site
of treatment and the choice of technique, if this is thought appropriate, and, second, to monitor the results of treatment.

Signs are to be sought segmentally, both anteriorly and posteriorly. The responsible vertebral level is sought by both palpation
and deep pressure techniques.

Palpation

Palpation is the key to osteopathic diagnosis on three counts:

(1) modification in the position of spinous and transverse processes,

(2) modification of intervertebral mobility, and

(3) modification of paravertebral tissues.

The first is unacceptable because vertebrae, like noses, vary a good
deal in shape and size. Second, the thickness of the muscles overlying
the transverse processes make the detection of the minimal difference
dividing the normal from the abnormal entirely subjective.

The second is also unacceptable because it too is wholly subjective
and there are distorting elements in that alterations in paravertebral

tissues confuse the sense of mobility obtained. The work of Hilton[7] and of Moll and Wright[8] throws further doubt on mobility as a diagnostic tool.

The third is fundamental to the system.

The palpatory techniques are four in number:

(1) 'skin drag',

(2) assessment of paravertebral muscle tone,

(3) 'skin rolling', and

(4) palpation for tenderness of muscles, attachment tissues etc.

Analysis of information obtained

The modifications found are due to:

(1) reflex paravertebral muscular contraction or inhibition

(2) periarticular reactions around an affected apophyseal joint

(3) tenderness which may be found widely distributed both anteriorly and posteriorly. Skin rolling is extremely useful here.

'Pressure' techniques

These are as follows.

(1) Springing. This simply shows a local abnormality, either of the vertebra itself or of the intervertebral joints, above or below.

(2) Lateral pressure to the spinous processes. This is a forced rotation, usually eliciting pain at the level already implicated by springing. It is also usually more painful in one direction than the other. This will indicate the manipulation intended, since this must be, in common sense, in the pain-free direction. This sign is clearly invalid in the cervical region, save for C7.

(3) Pressure over the apophyseal joints. This is sought at one finger's breadth from the spinous processes and is accurately named, as has been radiologically confirmed[91].

The various tests mentioned are described and illustrated in detail elsewhere in this text.

CONVENTIONAL RADIOLOGY

Before any detailed consideration of conventional radiology of the spine, it is important to identify the place of radiology in medical manipulation.

Conventional radiology is of importance when it can produce evidence not already to hand or not obtainable from other sources, and when that evidence may alter therapeutic decisions. The argument in favour of routine X-rays in practice is acceptable only as a defence against litigation, and is of dubious value to the patient, even slightly increasing the risk to the patient attendant upon any extraneous radiation. It is preferable that spinal X-rays be taken standing.

The indications for radiology are five.

(1) If the physician is not able to make a prediction from the patient's history and examination he may consider radiology as being potentially helpful, particularly in excluding pathological changes.

(2) If he fails therapeutically where he expects to succeed, he may find radiology helpful.

(3) If he has any suspicion of fracture, or of major pathological states, such as inflammatory arthritis or neoplasm.

(4) If the patient requests X-rays, he will be foolish not to concur.

(5) If there are known to be legal or insurance aspects to the case, the physician will need radiological support for his views, however unnecessary he may feel this to be from a clinical point of view.

X-rays taken for any of the first three indications are important because they may be of clinical value. Those taken at the request of the patient are likely to be of value mainly in reassuring the patient. Those taken for insurance or legal reasons are of greatest value in safeguarding the financial interests of the patient.

As to how radiological evidence may affect clinical decisions, this is primarily a question of whether or not to manipulate. The substantial majority of spinal problems seen in the practice of manual medicine are manipulable. It is important not to forget that gross changes on X-rays are easy to pick up, while it is the early changes that may matter. Again, it is vital to bear in mind that the opinion of a specialist radiologist may be necessary to determine whether a particular appearance is abnormal, or not.

It is crucial that the physician reporting on the radiographs is fully appraised of the clinical state of the patient. A normal X-ray by no means indicates that the patient has not pain of vertebral origin. The demonstration of quite marked degenerative changes occurs more commonly than not in a spine that is symptom-free. Congenital abnormality may be productive of symptoms, but this is not decided radiologically. Rheumatoid arthritis, the seronegative arthritides and neoplasm may not be radiologically demonstrable for a considerable period of time following their onset.

For those who see their own X-rays, the best way to avoid missing significant radiological signs must be to search each picture in the same routine sequence, and to this end a manipulative medicine method must be evolved and followed.

(1)   Identify the patient, the part and the date

(2)   Observe posture
    (a)   in the AP view
        (i)   rotation
        (ii)   lateral flexion
        (iii)   scoliosis

    (b)   in the lateral
        (i)   erect
        (ii)   in extension
        (iii)   in flexion
        (iv)   spondylolisthesis

(3)   Observe congenital defects
    (a)   cervical ribs
    (b)   defects of pars interarticularis
    (c)   spina bifida
    (d)   sacralization of L5

(4)   Intervertebral spaces
reduced in degenerative changes and disc disease

(5) Sclerosis of bone
   in degenerative disease, rheumatoid arthritis and late tuberculosis

(6) Osteophyte formation
   in degenerative disease, affecting intervertebral joints and apophyseal joints, encroaching on the foramina

(7) Porosis
   (a) general – senile etc,
   (b) localized – carcinoma, tuberculosis etc.,

(8) Cortical breaches
   (a) carcinoma
   (b) sarcoma
   (c) Scheuermann's disease
   (d) rheumatoid arthritis and allied conditions

(9) Interpedicular expansion
   intramedullary tumours

In summary, the manipulative physician must be clear in his own mind why he has ordered X-rays, and he must remain aware of the fact that radiological changes, like all disease processes, develop over a period of time. He must learn to recognize the slight signs of early change, and he must always be ready to seek expert advice, if he is not quite certain as to what he sees. Finally, he must guard against the temptation to use radiological evidence as an alternative to adequate history taking and thorough clinical examination.

POSTURE AND PROPHYLAXIS

It is common to think of the spine as an orthopaedic entity, and to forget its physiological role – that is, in movement, posture and proprioception. Wyke in 1970 showed that stimulating spinal joint nociceptors involved changes not only in muscle but also in the cardiovascular and respiratory systems[3]. Similarly, Dee in 1969 showed that moving one hip caused widespread muscle changes bilaterally[93]. It is clear that any movement has widespread consequences, including, of course, manipulation. Posture may be temporary, as in sleep. It may be fixed, as in pelvic tilt. It may be dynamic. Thus Roaf in 1978 defines it as 'the position the body assumes in preparation for the next movement'[94]. Posture is seen as a complex issue and almost quasiacademic, yet it is clinically significant in history taking, examination, treatment and, above all, prophylaxis.

In taking a history, we are not only interested in the distribution, nature and behaviour of pain, but also in the activities of daily living. These are of assistance in making an assessment and monitoring progress. Occupations as different as those of telephonist, typist or farmer obviously involve different postural problems. It must be remembered also that any posture maintained over a period of time can cause pain. Occupations requiring changes in position have a lower incidence of low back pain than those that do not[14].

It is a fact that those who drive a car every day are twice as likely to get back pain due to a prolapsed intervertebral disc as are those who do not, and that those who drive a car as part of their occupation are three times as likely to suffer back pain in comparison with non-drivers[15].

In examination, posture is clinically significant, as in the identification of kyphosis, scoliosis, muscle spasm or pelvic tilt. Pelvic tilt is traditionally regarded as of importance because of the system of osteopathic diagnosis, which is based on the theory that movements taking place at the sacro-iliac joints are principally or exclusively rotatory, and that pelvic asymmetry reflects this and denotes clinical abnormality. The movements taking place at the sacro-iliac joints are dealt with in detail in the summary on the pelvis (Chapter 4), but suffice it to say that rotation is only one of the several movements taking place at this complex joint. With regard to asymmetry, this presents practical difficulties because we are talking not of precise bony points but almost of anatomical neighbourhoods. Nicholls in 1960 wrote that 'the smaller the unit of measurement, the greater the incidence, and the larger the unit of measurement the greater the agreement'[95]. Pelvic tilt is still of clinical value because in a variable and unpredictable proportion of cases a heel raise can relieve symptoms.

The biofeedback principle has been employed in postural re-education. This involves a verbal stimulus being used to provide a kind of psychosomatic self-regulation. As early as 1900, in Germany, a system of autogenic training was established[96]. This is the basis of the Alexander exercises, devised in 1932[97]. In 1948 Barlow published work on 'postural homeostasis', whereby feedback from eyes, muscles and larynx could lead to 'postural re-education'[98]. Subsequently, both electrical and auditory signals have been used for the same purpose, particularly in the treatment of muscle spasm, and the use of electromyography is becoming very popular in this connection. But Reading[99], in a review in 1977, pointed out that results are conflicting, and in 1980 Hurrell wrote, 'few studies have been conducted with the rigour normally expected in clinical trials'[100]. Therefore, the value of biofeedback is still open to question.

In considering the role of posture in prophylaxis, we must exclude the single episode of back pain. In recurrent or persistent problems, however, it is of significance, and a simple system is to review resting posture, activities and preventative exercises. With regard to the cervical spine, let us consider the resting posture. Extension of the neck can pull on cervicobrachial nerve roots[101]. On the other hand, flexion can pull on the cervical roots and sleeves[102] and osteophytic bone can be pressed against the spinal cord[103]. Therefore, the best resting posture for the neck must be neutral position, with support if need be in the evening, or possibly the use of a soft collar, in particular in cases with morning pain. With regard to activity, any activity producing pain if persisted in should be curtailed. This is particularly relevant with regard to modification of work habit. Thus typists who develop discomfort or pain as the day wears on should be advised to 'walk it off' the moment discomfort appears. Carrying luggage is also a frequent source of neck pain, and should be avoided if possible; if avoidance is not possible the load should be evenly divided between the two hands. Driving is particularly hard on necks; collars should never be worn on driving, since they distort cervical proprioceptive reflexes and road traffic accidents can result[4]. On the advent of discomfort or pain, the driver should be encouraged to stop his car and to walk about for a few minutes.

With regard to the thoracic spine, ideal resting posture is lying on the floor, with the knees bent and a pillow under the head. Activities adversely affecting the thoracic spine are those such as hanging out washing or curtains, pushing motor cars or mowing lawns, and advice with regard to the curtailment of these activities should be given. The ideal angle for the trunk in driving is 120°, according to Andersson in 1974[104]. The ideal preventative exercise for the office worker with increasing pain or discomfort is to walk about the moment the symptoms appear.

With regard to the low back, the fog of war descends. Traditionally, the tendency to make a single diagnosis for all cases of back pain has led to restricted postural advice, stressing either kyphosis[105] or lordosis[106]. However, Nachemson in 1976 wrote, 'we do not know where the pain comes from, or at what level we are treating the patient, i.e. at the level of the motion segment, at the level of the dorsal horn neurone in the spinal cord, or at higher levels in the brain'[107]. All are now agreed that back pain is multifactorial in origin. Thus Weinstein in 1977 showed that both stenosis and lordosis were causes of pain[108]. Hutton and Adams in 1980 were able to show that both flexion and extension can be factors in the causation of pain and of degeneration of the spine[109]. It is noteworthy how recent this work is. Another myth, sadly, is that concerning the value of training in lifting. Wood showed that, between 1961 and 1967, there was an increase in episodes of back pain of 22%, and in duration of attack of 30%[110] – this at a time when training and advice with regard to lifting was widely available. Troup in 1979 came to the conclusion that 'there is little evidence based on prospective epidemiological studies to prove the value of training but there is no doubt that a well prepared programme can have satisfactory results, even if one of the mechanisms is the Hawthorn effect'[111]. The Hawthorn effect is that whereby any change of management produces an initial improvement, which is not maintained. Davis and Troup in 1966 have shown that such training was only of value in conditions similar to the laboratory and was not possible to obtain in real life[112]. Therefore, rigidity of advice and instruction with regard to low back pain is inappropriate, and pragmatism is what counts.

What matters with regard to hard or soft chairs or beds is what works. Since we know there is no one cause of back pain, no one posture or resting posture will be helpful in each and every case. With regard to advice concerning stooping or reaching, the best advice is the simplest: that is that the patient should close in on the work and lift at waist height. The nature of advice therefore should be undogmatic and uncomplicated. Above all, it should involve the patient, in that the patient should be invited to think out those positions and activities which are likely to prove harmful, and be encouraged to adjust his daily living accordingly.

SPONDYLOLISTHESIS AND SPINAL STENOSIS

The term 'spondylolisthesis' means the forward slip of a vertebral body on its subjacent fellow, this being secondary to a defect in the pars interarticularis. The incidence of the condition in the general population is not known, but it is frequently picked up radiologically and is often symptomless. It is not possible to give an accurate estimate of the percentage of all cases that do experience pain. In 1963, Newman, on the basis of changes observed in 319 cases, classified spondylolisthesis as follows[113]:

(1) congenital (66 cases)

(2) isthmic – this being due to a fatigue fracture of the pars interarticularis; or to the elongation of the pars interarticularis without bony discontinuity (164 cases)

(3) degenerative (80 cases)

(4) traumatic (three cases)

(5) pathological (six cases)

The severity of the slip is expressed in quarters of the sagittal dimension of the vertebral body. Thus the slip equal to half the sagittal diameter is a second degree listhesis and a three quarter displacement is a third degree slip.

Group 1 occurs at the L5/S1 segment and may cause secondary degenerative change. Group 2 is the commonest and the 5th lumbar segment is most commonly affected. Familial susceptibility has been established, and the factor of heavy and repeated occupational stress during particular postures also has been shown to be of importance. Group 3 is four times more common in females than in males, occurs most frequently at the L4/L5 level and is the type most often associated with nerve root involvement. The degenerative consequences for other elements of the mobile segment in the presence of this condition are obvious.

Spinal stenosis is a condition which has been neglected in the past. 'For nearly twenty years, the syndrome was confused with that of the protruded disc. Medical opinion to the contrary was either disregarded or unpublished'[108]. The term is used to denote the narrowing in the spinal canal but the shape is also significant, a narrow spinal canal of trefoil shape being a combination putting nerve roots at risk. It has been classified as being developmental and acquired. Acquired stenosis has been further subdivided into types:

Type 1   Degenerative change

(a)   posterior and posterolateral disc herniation and prolapse
(b)   massive central disc protrusion
(c)   ligamentum flavum thickening
(d)   posterior vertebral lipping
(e)   thickening of the neural arches
(f)   zygoapophyseal joint arthrosis
(g)   group 3 spondylolisthesis
(h)   isolated disc resorption

Type 2   Groups 1 and 2 spondylolisthesis

Type 3   Space-occupying new growths

Type 4   Paget's disease

Type 5   Iatrogenic disease following surgery

Type 6   Venous congestion

In view of Hitselburger's finding of 37% of abnormal myelographic appearances in 300 asymptomatic subjects, the condition is clearly very common[114]. Its study has been much enhanced by the work with ultrasound by Porter[115]. This has considerable clinical significance. For example, if the measurement is above the mean, the cause of back pain may not be in the canal at all. It may help to raise the question of whether the backache is mechanical, or if the lesion is in the root canal. Detection of this condition will also help surgeons to plan operations. Thus a very narrow canal is likely to incline him to decompress the canal by removing the laminae and spinous processes. It also helps detect the kind of spine which is likely to develop iatrogenic stenosis, and is a means of detecting spondylolisthesis when this is not always radiologically possible. Finally, it can be used to identify the kind of subject at risk and, if this is done, he can be offered vocational advice and also advice about the care of his back.

These conditions can clearly play a part in 'degenerative spondylosis'. To quote Vernon-Roberts: 'The initial event is a structural derangement of the intervertebral disc arising from the normal age-ing process, degeneration or prolapse. This is followed by a localized or generalized thinning of the disc with consequent forward tilting of the upper vertebral body resulting in antero-lateral bulging of the annulus and stimulation of marginal osteophyte formation. The abnormal stresses placed upon the apophyseal joints lead to bone remodelling and in some instances true osteo-arthrosis. Finally, alone or together, each of these pathological changes contributes to changing the mechanics of the spine at the level of the affected disc or discs'[116]. This condition has now been shown to be even more common than can be demonstrated radiologically. A recent study of 100 lumbar spines has shown that degenerative changes are present in the intervertebral discs of all subjects by middle age and are present in many spines by the age of 30. Since so many structures are involved in this process, it is difficult to identify the source of pain. Moreover, since the incidence of pain is far lower than uni-versal in ageing spines, the correlation of degenerative change with low back pain is a matter of conjecture. Therefore, the current com-mon practice of assuring a middle-aged patient with back pain that, in view of radiological changes demonstrated, his condition is fixed and immutable does not seem reasonable.

RHEUMATOLOGY AND ORTHOPAEDICS

Inflammatory conditions are encountered surprisingly rarely. This makes it all the more important to be conscious of them, as otherwise significant mistakes will be made.

Rheumatoid arthritis

The commonest inflammatory condition presents typically with pos-itive Rose–Waaler and latex tests, a raised erythrocyte sedimentation rate and 'erosive' X-ray changes. Manipulation has no place in the treatment of this disease. In the active phase, it would be pointless and painful. In the quiescent phase manipulation of the neck, with the possibility of jamming the odontoid process into the spinal cord, is potentially fatal and absolutely contraindicated.

The seronegative arthritides

Reiter's disease, psoriatic and colitic arthritides present little diag-nostic difficulty. Ankylosing spondylitis does, as its onset is fre-quently insidious and, in 75% of cases, presents with low back pain. Careful examination of the spine is essential – restriction of move-ment, notably of rotation of the dorsal spine, and a diminishing respiratory excursion in the young male being significant. These may be associated with iritis, aortic incompetence or colitic symptoms. The essential investigative finding is radiological evidence of sacro-iliitis. Diagnosis is important, as a policy of maximum mobility and full activity seems to affect the prognosis and ultimate restriction of movement markedly for the better. Manipulation in the active phase has no place and the clinician may miss the diagnosis. In the quies-cent phase manipulation is indicated where it is thought appropriate. The *'forme fruste'* of this disease is discussed below, in the section on Drug Treatment.

Scheuermann's disease

This is equally common in the two sexes. It usually presents between ages 13 and 17 with poor posture and aching in the region of the kyphosis, accentuated by standing and relieved by lying down. The kyphosis is thoracic in 75% of cases and thoracolumbar in 24%, and rarely purely lumbar. The thoracic cases present with accentuated dorsal kyphosis and increased lumbar lordosis. The thoracolumbar cases present with a long kyphosis and a short lumbar lordosis. Initially, the defect can be cured, but after 6–9 months it becomes fixed. There may be a local tenderness but there are no other marked physical signs.

In the active phase in severe cases results using a Milwaukee splint for a year are excellent, therefore early diagnosis of this not uncom-mon condition is important. Whereas manipulation in the active phase is useless and may delay diagnosis it can be of service in the quiescent phase, given appropriate indications. Mild cases frequently elude diagnosis, and it is common to find radiological evidence of Scheuermann's disease in adults who give no history of symptoms in adolescence.

Polymyalgia rheumatica

This is a rare condition that can readily mislead the medical manipulator. Presenting in the elderly with a history of marked early-morning stiffness and 'girdle' pain, it may be seen by the clinician when this has diminished. Signs are rare and the pain and stiffness may lead him to feel that manipulation may be of help. This is a potentially disastrous error. Thrombosis of the retinal artery is a feature of the condition and hence, blindness. The action to be taken is to take blood to estimate the erythrocyte sedimentation rate and start treatment with steroids immediately.

Osteoarthrosis

This condition is exceedingly common, indeed Vernon-Roberts has shown that by the age of 40 all discs show degenerative changes to a greater or lesser degree[116]. The condition, however, tends to be symptomatically episodic. In appropriate cases, manipulation plays a useful role.

Surgical referral

The proportion of cases we meet that require surgical referral is very small, but those that need it are serious and occasionally critical. Therefore it is important that the medical manipulator should have a clear picture of the indications for surgical referral.

In general, surgical referral is required when symptoms and disability the patient suffers are serious, prolonged or recurrent and do not respond to conservative treatment. Deterioration of symptoms despite treatment is another indication, particularly if neurological signs worsen.

The indications for referral are as follows.

(1) *Cervical spine:*
    (a) instability of the craniovertebral joint
    (b) persistent symptoms of vascular insufficiency particularly drop attacks, vertigo, tinnitus, etc
    (c) intractable and persistent unilateral neck and arm pain, resistant to other treatment

(d)   evidence of cervical myelopathy

(e)   bilateral root pain and neurological deficit in the upper limbs

(2)   *Thoracic spine:*

(a)   thoracic myelopathy

(b)   instability of a thoracic segment which does not respond to treatment

(3)   *Lumbar spine:*

(a)   symptoms of saddle anaesthesia or sphincter disturbance are an indication for instant referral

(b)   failure of other methods of treatment to relieve severe pain with or without neurological signs in one or both limbs

(c)   increase in neurological involvement, despite other treatments

(d)   intermittent claudication, associated with low back pain

(e)   segmental instability other methods have not corrected

LAY MANIPULATORS

In 1874, Andrew Taylor Still, an American, first promulgated his theory that the great majority of disease was due to spinal maladjustment, and that this could be remedied by manipulation. He regarded orthodox medicine as fallacious and harmful. This attracted the instant and enduring hostility of the medical profession. In the USA, over the years, osteopaths moved closer to medicine, and this provoked the foundation of chiropractic in 1895, by Mr Palmer, a grocer, who advocated, as his followers still do, a fundamentalist view as to the value of manipulation in the treatment of organic disease.

In Britain, there are between 2000 and 3000 lay osteopaths. However, the register of osteopaths, whose members have undergone formal training, numbers only a few hundred. The vast majority receive a vague and often scanty training, and in many cases none at all. There are several hundred chiropractors at present, taught in a variety of different colleges, with widely differing ideas and emphases, united only in their belief as to the sovereign merit of manipulation as a therapy appropriate to a variety of organic diseases.

Manipulation is not a cult or a philosophy or system of medicine, but merely a therapeutic tool, however useful. That is, it must be placed in the setting of all the many other treatments available to patients with musculoskeletal problems: physiotherapy, anti-inflammatory agents, analgesic agents, numerous injection techniques and even, if necessary, surgery.

Given that these techniques are in general reasonably safe and often helpful, the lay manipulator probably provides his local community with a valuable service. However, in the case of the lay manipulator, the principal issue is as to whether these manoeuvres should be deployed. This seems to offer a painfully restricted set of therapeutic options.

The medical manipulator should be trained in these techniques, with experience in orthopaedic or rheumatological practice, and have a special interest in and knowledge of osteoarticular neurology. This would seem to offer the patient greater security and place a wider range of diagnostic and therapeutic choices at his disposal.

This may seem reasonable and desirable, but it remains as yet an ideal. The reality is that the likelihood of the average member of the public receiving this form of treatment at the hands of medically qualified personnel is remote at the present time. Having said that, osteopathy and chiropractic quite rightly are of considerable interest to doctors, physiotherapists and others concerned with musculoskeletal disorders.

Lay manipulators have also made several contributions which should be acknowledged. Osteopaths were the first to suggest that a local examination of the spine, using palpatory and pressure techniques, was of value. This is becoming more widespread in medical practice, notably among those interested in spinal joint problems and their treatment by injection. Nevertheless, this is still not routine medical training. It seems a pity not to attempt to identify the level of a disorder, as this may help with the diagnosis. It may also indicate to which area the appropriate treatment should be directed.

Osteopathic theory was evolved since it was thought that all disease was due to vertebral displacement and could be cured by manipulation. Most of the several thousand osteopaths working today, however, would hold that vertebral problems had some aetiological connection with organic diseases and that treatment of the spine could influence these. There is no evidence to support this view.

It is also to the osteopath that we owe the most comprehensive codification of techniques, all aimed at achieving their object with minimum force.

THE DRUG TREATMENT OF MUSCULOSKELETAL PROBLEMS

Huskisson, in 1974, wrote: 'The clinician choosing a drug for his rheumatic patient is presented with a bewildering array of analgesic, anti-inflammatory, immuno-suppressive and other medicines. The same drug also appears under different names in different dosages, combinations and formulations'[117]. Carson Dick, in 1978, writes of this 'tidal wave of anti-rheumatic drugs' and suggests that clinicians faced with this choice should endeavour to use the minimum number of drugs possible in order to reduce confusion, and use the minimum amount of any single drug that achieves its therapeutic objective[118]. Lee et al., in 1974, noted that present-day prescribing habits leave much to be desired[119]. With regard to the mode of action of anti-rheumatic drugs, 'no unifying hypothesis currently in existence explains with any conviction why a variety of antirheumatic drugs work and, in particular, there is a dearth of evidence suggesting any degree of specificity'[120]. These drugs have widespread biological effects involving intracellular enzyme systems, membrane function and effects on mediators. 'In fact, none of the known biological effects of anti-rheumatic drugs can be produced in support of any existing theory which would explain why these drugs relieve the symptoms of many thousands of patients'[118].

Aspirin remains, after a century, the most commonly used drug with over 4000 million tablets being prescribed in the UK per annum. It is regarded as being well-tried and effective but, sadly, has a number of significant side-effects. Thirty per cent of patients on high-dose aspirin therapy have dyspepsia. Over 70% of people taking high-dose aspirin will suffer from gastrointestinal bleeding which, although in the great majority slight, will continue as long as they take the drug[121]. A connection between aspirin dosage and peptic ulceration has also been shown[122]. Nevertheless, 'aspirin is an effective anti-rheumatic drug which produces a wide range of biological effects'[118]. Another preparation which has been much studied is

47

indomethacin. It is regarded as an effective agent, particularly with respect to night pain[123]. Unfortunately, it also has side-effects which will involve about one third of the persons taking it. Dyspepsia is the most common and because of its association with haemorrhage and ulceration[124], it should not be prescribed for patients with peptic ulcers. The other major side-effects described by the authors of the papers cited here are such central nervous system symptoms as headaches and 'muzziness'. Other drugs include propionic acid derivatives, such as Brufen, Froben, Orudis, Fenopren and Naprosyn. Fenamates, such as Ponstan, are also available but Flenac has recently been withdrawn. With regard to pyrazolones, Butazolidine has also been withdrawn from prescription in general practice. With regard to the remaining preparations, insufficient information concerning their side-effects and clinical efficacy is available, making their comprehensive evaluation impossible at the present time. Analgesics such as Fortal, codeine phosphate, Distalgesic and paracetamol may be helpful. Occasionally, in cases of exceptionally severe pain, narcotic analgesics may be required. The prescription of oral steroids and such preparations as penicillamine and gold are decisions reserved for the rheumatologist.

The principal difficulty is to know when to deploy a particular drug out of this large variety, given our problems in establishing a valid diagnosis and our lack of understanding as to how they work. Jayson (1982) suggests that the history may be of help in this respect[125]. Those who suffer night pain and morning aching and stiffness which takes some time to work off, and who are then relatively symptom-free, are felt to have an inflammatory component to their disability. This has been highlighted by the discovery of HLA-B27, and its association with ankylosing spondylitis. According to Calin and Fries (1975), 2% of the population may suffer symptoms related to a 'forme fruste' of ankylosing spondylitis, which is a far higher figure than has been previously supposed[126]. In patients under the age of 40, having the symptoms described above, anti-inflammatory drugs may be strikingly effective.

In Jayson's view, another group of patients gets relief from pain on resting, while their symptoms are brought on again by movement and exercise. This group is probably suffering pain of primarily mechanical origin, and therefore analgesics are the drugs of choice for them. Nevertheless, in the absence of a more detailed understanding of the pathophysiology of back pain, the choice of drug, as every general practitioner knows, must remain largely empirical.

In view of the fact that the prescription of antirheumatic drugs is the principal therapeutic weapon deployed currently in hospital and in general practice, it is of interest that 'the mode of action of antirheumatic drugs is completely unknown, and too often authorities have produced evidence "validating" a particular mechanism, rather than attempting to find evidence which is discordant'[118]. The fact that the mode of action of antirheumatic drugs remains 'completely unknown' may surprise many clinicians. In view of this, the case for therapeutic empiricism in musculoskeletal disorders is strong.

COLLARS AND CORSETS

It is undeniable that elaborate collars will restrain movement of the neck in such cases as craniovertebral instability due to advanced rheumatoid arthritis. Aside from this group, however, it must be pointed out that the mode of action – if any – of collars is simply not known. There is no information with regard to their function available at all. Therefore, the varying and conflicting indications for their use that exist today are entirely based on supposition. When we turn to corsets, about which some information is now available, it will be seen that some assumptions made about corsets have been ill-founded. This is also likely to be the case with collars. Grieve says that the first principle in supplying a collar is 'never supply a cervical support without a plan to eliminate it'[45]. This is common sense. One point about collars is that if they are prescribed, certain advice must be given to patients, otherwise serious injury may ensue. Wyke, in 1965, demonstrated the importance of cervical mechanoceptors in governing the degree of dexterity in performing manual operations and in balance[127]. Lee and Lishman in 1975, have demonstrated the importance of vision in balance[128]. If a collar is prescribed, this will distort the cervical mechanoceptors and, therefore, the patient will rely almost entirely on vision. Such patients must be warned not to enter a dark room suddenly, as otherwise they risk accident. Furthermore, because of this distortion of the mechanoceptors in the neck, such patients wearing collars should be warned not to drive, as serious road traffic accidents have been recorded as a consequence[4].

With regard to corsets, the degree of confusion that exists may be indicated by the fact that in 1970, Perry described more than 30 different designs[129]. Nevertheless, more information is to hand than with regard to collars and some of this is disconcerting. For example Nachemson and Lindh, in 1969, proved that wearing a lumbar support for up to 5 years does not 'weaken the muscles'[130]. This conclusion was arrived at by a study of motor unit activity. Walters and Norris, in 1970, showed that there was no effect on lumbar musculature during standing and slow walking, but during fast walking the support actually increased muscle activity[131]. Van Leuven and Troupe, in 1979, showed the range of sagittal movement was the same whether a healthy symptom-free subject wore an instant corset, a tailored lumbar corset or no support at all[132]. Thus, elaborate corsets may make some movements uncomfortable but it does little to prevent them. Norton and Brown, in 1957, inserting Kirschner wires into the lumbar spinous processes of a normal subject, found that commonly-used low back braces and plaster-of-Paris jackets failed to limit lumbar movements[133]. These actually appeared to increase lumbosacral movement by restricting motion in the rest of the spine. Hence, the basis of the prescription of corsets for many years, i.e. that it limited spinal movement, is shown to be untrue. Further, Nachemson, in 1964, found that a tight lumbar support reduced intradiscal pressures by about 30%[134]. This has led Macnab in 1977 to write, 'the most important component of the spinal brace is the abdominal binder'[43]. This evidence has led to the increasing popularity of abdominal strengthening exercises in the treatment of low back pain. This is certainly reasonable, but as to how effective these exercises are, there is as yet no evidence.

TRACTION

Traction, as a form of therapy, is as ancient as manipulation. Its value has never been proven, nor the way it works understood. It certainly involves mechanoceptor stimulation. 'I suspect it may provide transitory relief of pain by stimulating receptors'[125]. It has been claimed that it will reduce disc protrusion. 'There remains no evidence to suggest ... that actual disc protrusion can be reduced by this means'[41]. De Sèze showed that, with high poundages, the L4/5 space can be increased by 1.5 mm and the L3/4 space by as much as 2 mm[135]. However, the spaces return to their pre-traction level, either on release from traction, or on standing up. Nachemson showed that pulls of half of a normal subject's body weight will increase lumbar vertebral spaces by 1.5 mm and the intradiscal pressure by up to 25%[136]. In a study on the value of traction, Matthews demonstrated separation of vertebral bodies and increased centripetal forces exerted by the tension applied to the surrounding soft tissues[137]. He found, however, that it produced no detectable advantage over other treatments.

A typical trial was one by Weber in Oslo, on patients described as having disc prolapse[139]. The criteria for this were sciatica, neurological deficit and positive myelographic signs. Thirty-seven patients with these symptoms and signs were compared with a control group of 35 treated by simulated traction, and there was no significant difference in treatment results between the two groups. However, it is now known that 37% of people with positive myelograms are pain-free and Mooney has shown clearly that the traditional neurological examination is not entirely reliable[52]. Further, it is now accepted that the causes of leg pain are many, so that few people nowadays would accept that the 72 patients concerned either had prolapsed discs or even the same cause for their symptoms and signs. Again, we have very little evidence of the precise diagnosis of the cause of pain in this series. Under these circumstances, it is virtually meaningless to attempt to assess any form of treatment in this way.

'In the absence of a valid diagnosis, controlled therapy is not possible'[4].

In this sense, the situation with regard to traction is analogous to that of manipulation. Traction is harmless and empirical. Every physiotherapist knows that it has its successes as well as its failures, and it seems unreasonable to deny its use to a patient because we do not know the diagnosis, and when he may yet benefit from such therapy.

For the general practitioner, traction may prove of great value. It is not widely known that this is the case, but a number of different apparatuses exist, suitable for use in the surgery or the patient's home. This is true of both cervical and lumbar traction.

Cervical traction is of value in cases where manipulation has failed, or where it is likely to be painful or is otherwise contraindicated. Particularly, it is useful in the ageing neck, with marked degenerative change giving rise to brachial symptoms. In this case, it must be combined with appropriate exercises. It may be applied manually, either sustained or rhythmic, or it may be applied mechanically.

The simplest unit for use in the home comprises a steel spreader bar, so designed that it is strong but light, which is suspended from a suitable hook in the patient's home. This latter must be securely fixed, in particular *not* to a banister. The head harness consists of two webbing pieces, one for the chin, the other for the occiput, freely running on two nylon cords.

Lumbar traction may be useful in cases where manipulation or other treatments have failed in patients with low back or leg pain.

Use of a domestic traction apparatus has certain practical advantages for the patient. There is no wait for therapy. There is no waste of patient time in travelling. Therapy may be adjusted to the patient's domestic and occupational needs.

An example of such an apparatus is described and illustrated in Chapter 11.

EXERCISE AND EXERCISES

In this area, as in many others in this field, the degree of confusion that exists is extraordinary, and it is of interest to try to establish the reality, in contradistinction to conjecture. The correlation between physical fitness and the incidence of low back pain is far from clear. Bergquist-Ullman and Larsson found little difference in the incidence of low back pain between office workers and manual workers[12]. However, manual workers suffered a significantly longer period of disability, both in the initial episode and in recurrences. Cady *et al.* studied a large number of Los Angeles firemen, and discovered that physical fitness in a series of nearly two thousand cases had a significant preventative effect on the incidence of back injuries[31]. However, in the same study, it was found that, not only did the two groups differ from the point of view of physical fitness, but in other ways as well, so that it was difficult to determine whether the reduction of incidence of back pain was due to relative fitness or to some other, linked factor. 'Difficulties in measuring back and abdominal muscle strength and subject selection make the assessment of possible correlations difficult'[16]. Thus the correlation between fitness and the prevention of back pain, which has been assumed by many to be a real factor, while it still may be true, is not proven.

Keyserling *et al.* used pre-employment strength testing procedures and found that the risk of back injury increased threefold when the job requirement exceeded the strength capability on an isometric simulation of the job[139]. These findings may be relevant to the prescription of exercises. Thus, 'it remains to be shown that strong muscles protect the back from painful episodes, and no evidence has been presented to suggest that subjects with low back pain possess particularly weak back muscles'[140].

Despite the above, exercises are probably the most commonly prescribed physical remedy, world wide, certainly as far as rheumatologists and orthopaedic surgeons are concerned (*see* reference 140). Recent work has altered attitudes as to which exercises are appropriate. Professor Jayson wrote, 'In my own view, the right sort of exercises for most back pain patients are isometric exercises, aimed at strengthening the paraspinal and abdominal muscles'[125]. Nachemson, over 20 years' measuring intradiscal pressures in the lumbar spine, has shown that some exercises increase the load on the lumbar spine to such an extent that the intradiscal pressures reach levels as high as those measured in standing and leaning forwards with weights in the hands[141]. Particularly marked is this rise in sitting-up exercises, with the knees either flexed or extended. Therefore, it must be accepted that these should be avoided, which is one of the reasons why isometric exercises are currently in favour.

Nachemson's figures for intradiscal pressures at L3-4 in subjects show a load of 70 kg on standing; on bilateral straight leg raising of 120 kg; on sitting-up exercises, knees flexed and extended, of 180 and 175 kg respectively; and on isometric abdominal muscle exercises of 110 kg[141].

It has been shown by Lindstrom and Zachrisson that these exercises, alone or in combination with traction, give better results than ordinary flexion and extension exercises[142]. Moreover, it is known that, when lifting or carrying very heavy objects, the increase of intra-abdominal pressure resulting from contraction of the abdominal, pelvic and costal muscles, and the diaphragm, will relieve some of the load on the lumbar spine. Therefore, it is 'reasonable' (Nachemson) to perform exercises aimed at strengthening these muscles[141]. A further function of exercises is psychological. They are now commonly undertaken by people with chronic back pain, and Fordyce wrote about operant conditioning and graded exercise programmes, which involve the patient in trying to reduce the severity and frequency of low back pain[143]. This points to part of the reason for the success of the low back pain school in Sweden, involving, as it does, patient explanation and exhortation[140].

VERTEBRAL INJECTIONS

These are increasingly used and have been the focus of much interesting work in the last 10 years. Their value is great and is becoming more and more established. No medical manipulator can afford to ignore them, and the fact that they are not available to the lay-manipulator must be as damaging as a lack of knowledge of articular neurology.

Materials used

Local steroids and anaesthetics alone, or in combination, and sometimes sclerosants, are employed.

Techniques

1. Injection of soft tissue trigger points

Non-articular rheumatism is an ill-defined phenomenon which is not understood. Nevertheless, it is a fact that patients with back and leg pain associated with tender 'fibrositic' areas in muscles and ligaments, or similar areas around an affected spinal joint, can have their symptoms relieved if these nodules are infiltrated with local anaesthetic.

'One of the most poorly understood phenomena related to the chronic pain syndromes is the focal hyper-irritability of tissues related to painful areas in the body. ... by a poorly understood mechanism local injections with anaesthetic provide pain relief at a distant location far longer than can be explained by the pharmacological action of the drug'[144]. This observation is supported by the work of Mehta in 1973[145].

2.   Peripheral nerve block

This technique has existed for more than a century[146]. While this form of treatment is frequently very effective, accurate needling is often difficult because of variations in the course of nerves, difficulties of detecting landmarks and obesity in some patients. The commonest nerve block employed by the generalist is that of the greater occipital nerve in intractable headache. It is of interest that Sunderland, in 1978, wrote, 'The biopsy specimens that I have had the opportunity of examining histologically have shown surprisingly little to account for the distressing pain associated with entrapment'[147].

3.   Injection of attachment tissues

The attachments of ligaments, muscles and aponeuroses are common sources of pain for reasons which are ill understood[50]. Their detection by detailed local examination and treatment by injection are well worthwhile[148]. Steroids and anaesthetics may be used in combination but pain relief from the anaesthetic may wear off after a few hours and the steroid may not begin to work for some days, although this is far from being invariably the case[144]. Nevertheless, the patient should be warned of this phenomenon. Examples of such problems which occur frequently are the various rotator cuff problems, tennis and golfer's elbow and the 2nd and 3rd costochondral junctions in Tietze's disease. In the lumbar region common sites are the inter- and supraspinous ligaments and tissue attachments along the iliac crest.

Ingpen and Burry had considerable success in combining one or two injections with lumbar isometric exercises[149]. They infiltrated the region of maximum tenderness between the L5 spinous process and the posterior superior iliac spine with a suspension of 1 ml of prednisolone acetate (25 mg per ml) and 2 ml of procaine hydrochloride (2%), with satisfactory results.

4. Zygoapophyseal injections

It is now realized that these joints are a common source of pain[52] and recent work has also raised neurological implications of great interest[144]. These injections are also eminently suitable for use in general practice and therefore (particularly in the lumbar region) they will be considered in some detail. Mooney injected 20 patients (15 with chronic low back pain, five normal) with irritant hypertonic saline[150]. This evoked marked myoelectrical activity in the hamstring muscles and limitation of straight leg raising to 70%. Three of the group had depressed deep tendon reflexes. This will be recalled when disc problems are discussed. All signs, including the reflexes, were restored to normal by a second injection of 2-5 ml of 1% Xylocaine. Further studies by this author suggest that 20% of low back pain sufferers obtain long-term relief through this technique, and a further one third, partial relief.

The dangers of these techniques in the upper cervical spine, including brainstem ischaemia and the sequelae of this phenomenon[151], will be discussed in detail in Chapter 2, in the section on Cervical Injections. This technique is *not* the same as injecting 'trigger points', since infiltrating soft tissues is different from depositing material into a synovial joint cavity.

5. Epidural local analgesia

This will be considered in detail in Chapter 4, in the section on Lumbar Injections. Suffice it to say, at this stage, that it has a considerable role to play in low back pain and sciatica of non-discal origin.

6. Sclerosant therapy

Substantial disagreement persists as to the mechanisms of action of sclerosants in this field. Considerable disagreement is also evident in respect of whether or not sclerosant therapy has a place in this field at all. Discussion will not be entered into at this stage.

ELECTRO-ACUPUNCTURE AND TRANSCUTANEOUS ELECTRICAL NERVE STIMULATION

These two therapies are considered together because, in the light of recent work, it seems likely that their modes of operation are closely allied, if not identical[53]. They are but two of a number of therapies employing peripheral stimulation for the relief of pain.

Classical acupuncture is a therapy of very long standing, and it is only of recent years that the mystery surrounding it has been tempered by studies, which, in Western orthodox medical eyes, have been based on scientifically acceptable principles[53]. By and large, these studies have confirmed the efficacy of acupuncture in the relief of many types of pain[53]. One matter of interest which has come to light in recent years is the correlation to be found between the acupuncture points for pain control and trigger points.

The more recent development of electro-acupuncture employs somewhat similar theories, but uses a low-frequency electrical pulse, instead of the purely mechanical stimulation of classical acupuncture needles. Here it is pertinent to be reminded of the fact that various injection techniques have been shown to have effects lasting very much longer than the known pharmacological action of the materials injected[144]. An increasing number of acupuncturists practise electro-acupuncture as an adjunct to classical acupuncture, using the needles as intramuscular electrodes. More commonly, however, electro-acupuncture is practised without invasion of the tissues.

The patient holds one electrode in his hand, while the physician holds the wandering electrode. The first stage is to identify an acupuncture point thought to be relevant to the patient's symptoms. This is done by moving the wandering electrode over the skin in the selected area, with the apparatus switched to 'constant', the intensity in mid-range, until such time as the indicator light is illuminated, with or without an accompanying 'bleep'. The volume is then adjusted so that the patient is aware of a sensation about the electrode before the mode is switched to 'pulsed'. The machine then delivers a pulsed signal, at a pause frequency of the physician's choice (within the range offered by the particular instrument). A number of such points may be treated at one session, for a few minutes each, the intensity being controlled by the patient's tolerance.

Too high an intensity results in quite sharp pricking in the area of his pain; too low an intensity is unfelt. The placing of the wandering electrode is critical, in that moving it away from an acupuncture point by as little as 2 mm commonly results in loss of signal. Clearly, the point is one where the impedance offered by the tissues between the electrodes is markedly reduced, so that it is tempting to assume that this anatomically well-defined point is related to the best electrical conductor in a man, a nerve. On this assumption, electrical stimulation of a nerve will activate the gate control system in the spinal cord. If the frequency and the intensity of the signal are suitable, the larger, more readily activated fibres of the mechanoceptors will play their part in provoking the endorphin release which inhibits the transmission of pain input from the smaller, less readily activated nociceptor fibres[4]. As in the case of other means of stimulating mechanoceptor input, and provided the stimulation of the mechanoceptor fibres is not accompanied by marked nociceptor stimulation, the greater the stimulation (within the limits of patient tolerance), the greater the pool of endorphin and thereby the better pain control.

There are numerous machines on the market. A typical example (small, battery operated and easily portable) gives a square curve oscillation between 25 milliseconds and 1 second, and a pulse frequency between the same limits. Maximum output is a modest 4 mA.

Transcutaneous electrical nerve stimulation is different, in that no attempt is made to pick up a point of cutaneous low impedance, but rather is a stream of electrical impulses applied between two skin electrodes, so placed as to direct those impulses in the region of a nerve related to the patient's symptoms. Thus it is of wider application, in that little skill is required, and it may readily be used by the patient in a domiciliary setting. The object is similar to that of electro-acupuncture, in that an attempt is made to stimulate the larger, mechanoceptor fibres in preference to the smaller, nociceptor fibres, thus causing the same inhibition of pain conduction.

Once again, there are many machines on the market. A typical example (weighing but a few ounces and readily carried in a pocket) gives a peaked curve oscillation from 0 to 100 Hz, with a pulse frequency between 1.5 ms and 1 s, and a power output up to 60 mA. Thus it is possible to vary the frequency of signal, the frequency of pulse trains and the intensity of signal over quite wide ranges, so as to produce maximum effect in different patients and at different sites. The question of topically lowered impedance does not arise.

The clinical application of either of these therapies is essentially twofold; (1) they are of value where other therapies have failed to relieve symptoms and (2) they are of value where manipulation is contraindicated, or where injections have been declined. TNS has the added advantage referred to, in being suitable for self-treatment by the patient. In this latter case, it is worth while teaching the patient how to use his machine, then giving him one on trial for a week or two, prior to his acquiring one of his own.

RHIZOTOMY AND RHIZOLYSIS

Rhizotomy, which is the cutting of nerve root or primary ramus, is not suitable for use in general practice. Nevertheless, it is of considerable clinical interest, because it throws light on the complexity of innervation of the various structures in the back, particularly of the paravertebral musculature and the apophyseal joints. The technique was pioneered by Rees, who used a tenotome for bilateral, subcutaneous, multiple rhizotomy[152]. He obtained a high success rate, and by 1971 over 3000 patients had been treated, no significant complications having been recorded. This technique was used by Toakley in 1973 on 200 cases, who had suffered back pain for an average of 9 years[153]. Results were good in 125 cases, fair in 37, improved in 36 and worse in two. It was later noted by Burnell, doing electromyographic (e.m.g.) work on patients who had undergone this treatment, that segments of paravertebral muscle had been denervated[154]. He felt that this might have been a factor in pain relief.

Subsequent X-ray investigation by King in 1977 showed that, due to the shortness of the blade in use, the tenotome of Rees had never reached the apophyseal joint capsule[155]. Therefore, presumably, the results had indeed been due to the denervation of paravertebral muscle, rather than rhizotomy. King then did a comparative study, using high frequency coagulation rhizolysis, directed to the apophyseal joint capsule. It is fascinating that the Rees method produced a 71% satisfactory result and the rhizolysis a 72% satisfactory result. The similarity of results lends force to the idea of a close neurological interrelationship between the structures directly affected by these different techniques. In one case in which there was evidence of a large extradural defect at the L4/15 level on myelography and weakness of the right hallucis longus, pain was relieved by this procedure and toe strength returned to normal. One is reminded of Mooney and Robertson's finding with regard to tendon reflexes[52]. In a further seven patients with positive radiology and back pain, six were

59

relieved completely after this treatment. Of the seven, only four required surgical intervention in the long term.

This led King to assert that, although backache and sciatica may be initiated by prolapse of the intervertebral disc, it can also be generated by a pain/muscle spasm cycle of structures innervated by the primary and posterior rami. The interruption of this neurological circuit may well relieve the symptoms. Oudenhoven, in 1979, in a group of 337 patients, achieved 83% excellent pain relief using this treatment[156]. Pain relief correlated directly with postoperative e.m.g. changes, and it was noted that unilateral denervation failed to control pain.

Thus, in the absence of effective denervation, pain control is poor and temporary. Moreover, structures in the apophyseal capsule clearly have contralateral as well as ipsilateral effects. This clinically confirms the experimental work of Wyke in 1970[3] and Dee in 1969[93]. King, in 1977, writes, 'It is difficult to escape the conclusion that structures innervated by the posterior primary rami play an important role in generating the back and leg pain which accompanies acute disc rupture'[155]. This is scarcely surprising when one considers how extraordinarily widely distributed are the nociceptive nerve endings in lumbosacral tissues, as has been discussed in the section on classification of back pain in Chapter 4, and the capacity that so many of these tissues have of generating muscle spasm, in addition to producing pain, on nociceptive stimulation. Thus, the work done on these treatments emphasizes the multifactorial nature of back pain and the difficulty of endeavouring to isolate a single causative factor.

SCLEROSANT THERAPY

Sclerosant therapy was first introduced into Britain by Barbor[157], based upon the earlier work of Hackett. Originally, the materials employed were phenol and zinc sulphate, which were aimed at the ligamento-periosteal junctions of ligaments described as 'insufficient'. In 1959, the commonly used material was changed to the less irritant mixture of dextrose, glycerine and phenol, which, as with the previous injection, was mixed with procaine. There has been evidence adduced demonstrating fibrosis and a proliferation of osteophytes at the site of injection[158].

Barbor advocates the use of sclerosant therapy in cases of lumbar 'instability'. Although clearly defined, lumbar instability is almost impossible to identify, in view of the work of Hilton, referred to above in the section on Spinal Mobility[7]. This must detract from the theoretical validity of the therapy, and the clinical indications cover a substantial number of possible diagnoses. Resolution of pain subsequent to treatment may arise from numerous factors other than that therapy; there is no clear correlation between treatment and its effect. However, Barbor's $27\frac{1}{2}\%$ crude failure rate is generally accepted by workers employing his method.

Nonetheless, sclerosant therapy is widely employed in this country, with results apparently reasonably favourable and, provided that the dextrose is not used in concentration greater than $12\frac{1}{2}\%$ (said to preclude the risk of local necrosis), the added pain transiently caused to the patient appears the only real disadvantage. A better understanding of the disease processes underlying 'ligamentous insufficiency' would help to rationalize this therapy. Neither of the authors employs this treatment.

ASSESSMENT OF RESULTS AND THE ASSOCIATED DIFFICULTIES

Assessment of results of manipulative therapy is difficult for two main reasons: first because of the subjective nature of the most important single criterion – pain, and second because the committed manipulator is denied the facility of the controlled trial on ethical grounds.

The reason for this denial is that he is forced to afford treatment to a proportion of his patients which, rightly or wrongly, he believes to be second best. A further substantial difficulty lies in the fact that it is seldom possible to make an accurate diagnosis, and that, as a result of this, it is difficult for treatment not to be empirical[4, 140].

There have been numerous attempts in the past to measure pain. All have suffered the same major disadvantage, in that they have required sophisticated or time-consuming procedures, which have rendered them unsuitable for employment in busy clinical practice. If it is possible to enlist the co-operation of a non-manipulator, then measurement of pain may be obviated by random selection of patients in a controlled, cross-over trial, it being reasonable to assume that variations in pain threshold and pain tolerance are similar in each randomly selected group of the sample. Success of the procedure is measured numerically in the proportion of each group expressing themselves pain-free, or substantially improved within defined time limits. Otherwise, it is necessary to accept crude evidence of the patient's statement of improvement.

It is also possible to observe changes in physical signs, in posture, in apparent differences in leg length, etc, which may be utilized in the overall assessment of results. There may be changes in the palpatory tests of Maigne and in the range and relative asymmetry of movements. There may be measurable improvement in performance of tasks and alteration in sleep pattern. Restriction of activities of daily living may be lessened, and some of these may be demonstrable by observation of the patient undressing, etc.

One of the oft-repeated criticisms of manipulation is the inherent danger attaching to this form of therapy. In fact, the dangers are few and very clearly defined, and these have been detailed above, in the section on Indications, Contraindications and Dangers. Disasters are of rare occurrence and are almost exclusively the result of ignoring a clear contraindication to manipulation, rather than to some manipulation being performed inexpertly. It seems likely that the success of manipulation by lay operators is a reflection of the simplicity of techniques suited to the task and the rarity of the conditions favouring disaster. Provided the contraindications already listed are faithfully observed, the bogey of danger may in practice be ignored.

As an example of reliance on the patient's statement of improvement in pain level, coupled with improvement in range of movement, the figures on pages 64 and 65 illustrate the results likely to be achieved by the manipulator engaged primarily in general practice. They are derived from a series of 1037 cases of vertebral pain, unselected except by virtue of the patient's choice of physician. Results are labelled good where the patient has declared himself free of pain and where the range of movement is as good or better than it was prior to therapy, moderate where mobility is substantially improved and severity of pain is reduced, and poor where there is no reported or observable improvement.

As it is impossible to measure pain objectively[159,160] the analysis of these results was deliberately crude (not employing statistical method), reliance being placed upon a large sample, upon a self-rating basis.

In the lumbar spine, the results to be expected are not so dramatic as in the cervical spine, but are still encouraging. The overall figure of 79% is made up of 36% in one session, 58% in two sessions and 66% in three.

For those whose inclination is towards research and the adduction of statistically sound evidence in support of their conclusions, the controlled trial offers a format well suited to the task and easily applied to this purpose, provided a non-manipulator, neutral or antagonistic, is available.

It is suggested that a small part of the field be selected for scrutiny (for example, cervical pain), and that a list of exclusions be agreed, in an attempt to eradicate unnecessary confusion arising from the influence of non-vertebral factors. A special clinic is opened, overtly research-based, either to which doctors are invited to send patients, or which patients are invited to attend. At the initial consultation, both clinicians see each patient, applying the agreed exclusion criteria, those patients so excluded being treated in an orthodox way and not included in the trial.

All patients selected for the trial are allotted to either clinician on a random basis, preferably by employing an independent statistician to prepare in advance sealed serially-numbered envelopes determining the choice of therapist.

Each clinician treats patients so referred to him in the manner he believes to be best for them, each patient being requested to fill in a simple questionnaire as to pain level, etc, on the third day of the trial, at the same time being given a follow-up appointment for one week, to which he brings his completed questionnaire.

At the end of the first week, improvement is recorded, together with the day of resolution of pain, those patients pain-free being discharged from the clinic. Those whose symptoms persist are seen again at the end of the second week, when, again, those who have become pain-free during the week are discharged from the clinic. At the end of the third week, those who have become pain-free during the previous week are discharged from the clinic, and those whose pain still persists are transferred to the other clinician, the whole process being repeated for the other half of the trial.

Assessment of results is made in two forms: first the proportion of each half sample gaining resolution of pain within 3 weeks is compared, then the time taken to achieve this, 3 days, 1 week, 2 weeks,

Therapy related to results and number of attendances in 364 cervical lesions

Therapy	Good					Moderate				
	1	2	3	4	5+	1	2	3	4	5+
Percentage of lesions	51·9	21·2	10·7	5·8	2·8	0·8	1·1	0·6	0·3	0·8
Manipulation	189	77	39	21	10	3	4	2	1	3
Suspension	1	3	4	1	1	0	0	0	1	1
Auto/susp.	0	0	1	0	1	0	0	0	0	0
Depo medrone	2	5	2	1	1	0	0	0	0	0
Other	2	0	2	0	0	0	0	0	2	1
Overall results	343 – 92·4%					17 – 3·6%				

Histogram   Percentages of total cervical lesions treated by manipulation

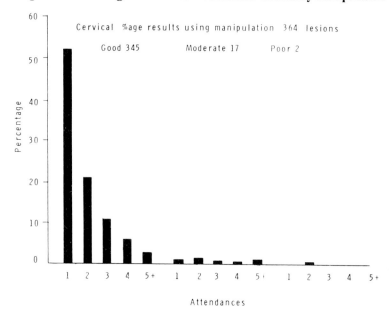

Therapy related to results and number of attendances in 768 lumbar lesions

Therapy	Good					Moderate				
	1	2	3	4	5+	1	2	3	4	5+
Percentage of lesions	36·3	21·9	8·1	4·7	8·5	2·1	1·2	1·3	1·2	2·5
Manipulation	279	168	62	36	65	16	9	10	9	19
Sust/traction	11	28	35	28	55	1	6	5	12	14
Dom/Traction	0	0	0	0	2	0	1	0	0	0
Epidural L.A.	6	8	4	4	13	1	1	2	3	3
Depo medrone	19	18	8	3	12	0	2	0	1	3
P$_2$G Sclerosant	4	1	2	1	4	0	0	0	3	4
Other	3	3	5	2	5	0	1	0	0	1
Overall results			689					72		
			79.5					8.3		

Histogram   Percentages of total lumbar lesions treated by manipulation

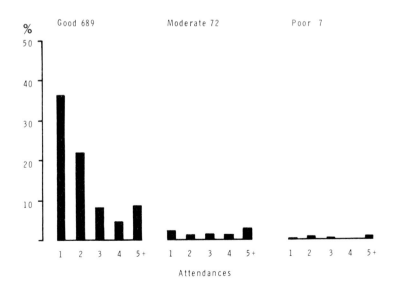

LUMBAR %AGE RESULTS USING MANIPULATION-768 LESIONS

65

or 3 weeks. Sudsidiary results may be derived from applying the same process to the second half of the trial, that concerning the 'failures' of the first half.

This is the basic form of trial, whereby results of medical manipulation may be compared with those of more generally accepted therapies (such as the use of a collar). If it is desired, comparison may be made between further, different therapies, thus adding to the complexity of the trial. But, however it is decided to conduct the trial, one essential to easing the task of analysis must be the manner in which data are recorded, and it must be appreciated that statistical analysis is very much the province of the computer.

It is quite possible to analyse results with pencil and paper; it is rather less time-consuming with a simple punched card system and a knitting needle, although this requires the prior design and production of record cards which, while simplifying the task of data extraction, limits the flexibility of analysis by virtue of the rigidity of its design. It is, however, a slow business with anything but small samples and simple data. The computer very largely eradicates the problem of inflexibility and is very much faster in operation, and it is well suited to anything but the most minor of trials.

The computer is no more than a manipulator of figures, however, and to obtain statistically significant results data must be fed into it in such a form as to be manipulable according to the design and capability of the particular instrument used. Just as good design of the punched card system is of equal importance to coding and entry of data, so writing a satisfactory program is fundamental to the efficient use of the computer. Much unnecessary work may be avoided by entering data in a form and sequence that are compatible with the program of instructions that is to be employed.

It was with this in mind that the data recording sheets were designed for history, examination and therapy. The computer program is written round these sheets in such a manner as permits both relatively simply input of material and rapid extraction of data in respect of particular features which may be found to be common to numerous patients. Thus, an individual patient's record may be entered, stored, recalled or amended, while factors of possible research interest may be recalled in relation to those patients who exhibit them. Accordingly, the computer is of value in both clinical record handling, and in research. Further, the administrative burden of appointments, accounts etc may be lightened, and efficiency established and maintained with reduced time and effort, by the employment of an administrative program.

One serious problem does, however, remain, in that in this field of medicine there is commonly no specific diagnosis, and therefore the value of statistical analysis of results is restricted to the comparison of efficacy of therapies for a whole group of conditions. Efficacy studies have but a modest place in the scientific evaluation of medical manipulation, and the more important area for research must lie in improving diagnosis and a better understanding of the mechanisms of therapy. It is in this field that the computer may best show its value.

The British Association of Manipulative Medicine, the International Federation of Manual Medicine, the British League Against Rheumatism and the Back Pain Association

The British Association of Manipulative Medicine (BAMM) was formed in 1963. This largely as a consequence of the realization that the not insignificant number of doctors practising a wide variety of manipulative techniques in the UK were isolated, without any means of pooling knowledge and aspirations.

The following year, as a result of similar trends in other countries, the Fédération Internationale de Médicine Manuelle (FIMM) was instituted, BAMM becoming affiliated to this new body as its official British representative. FIMM now embraces twenty-three member countries.

The constitution of BAMM sets out the prime objects of the Association as being the promotion of postgraduate education in this subspeciality of medicine and research in the science and art of manipulation. To these ends there has evolved a pattern of teaching over eight weekends, complemented by a follow-up weekend, spread over two winters, but no collective research of any consequence has yet been undertaken. The Association has built up a cadre of tutors who also take part in seminars at other meetings at various venues throughout the country. A few tutors have gone to the extent of offering independent courses in medical manipulation, and a number of members have published work in this field. The *Newsletter* serves to keep members in touch with events.

BAMM plays its part in the triennial congresses of FIMM, in 1983 being one of six member countries invited to make a formal presentation of the British school's work. It also plays a part in the administrative structure of FIMM, its President and Honorary Secretary being members of the General Assembly. Through the Honorary Secretary, BAMM is also currently represented on the Scientific Advisory Committee of FIMM.

BAMM admits to membership as an associate any registered medical practitioner who expresses an interest in medical manipulation. Full membership, currently being reviewed by a working party, is at present restricted to those largely (or exclusively) employed in this field, whose work and experience, following proposal and seconding by full members, is approved by Council of the Association.

In the past there has been no effort to coordinate teaching in different countries, but, in 1983, FIMM pioneered the first international workshop, in which BAMM played a full part. It is to be hoped that this will prove to be the springboard for much closer international cooperation than has hitherto obtained.

Happily, international cooperation is already on the increase, and this is a trend that can do nothing but good in the promotion of collaboration and the improvement of international standards. Part of this cooperation is reflected in the current attempt to produce a common nomenclature, a task of very substantial proportions. A further aspect lies in the tutor exchange pioneered by Britain, whereby senior tutors attend courses, either as observers or as demonstrators, and this trend is also to be seen in foreign students attending courses in different countries.

The British League Against Rheumatism (BLAR) is the 'umbrella' organization in the UK giving coherence to the activities of the numerous agencies devoted to tackling the many aspects of musculoskeletal problems. It is the official representative of this country in the European League Against Rheumatism.

BLAR has two main divisions: a Community Section, composed in the main of lay organizations and bodies involved in the social problems of rheumatic disorders in the community as a whole, and a Scientific Section, with a heavy preponderance of rheumatologists, playing a major role in coordinating and promoting rheumatological research in Britain.

Over the past few years an organization has emerged in Britain, which is unique in being the only body of lay origin exclusively devoted to the study of back pain and its relief. This is the Back Pain Association (BPA). In a relatively short period the BPA set up a Research Committee, manned largely by distinguished doctors, which studies and evaluates research projects submitted to it. BPA funds such research, if approved by the Research Committee.

The BPA has promoted one substantial international symposium and taken part in many others. It has also engaged itself in an advertising campaign in the pursuit of improved public understanding of the problems surrounding back pain. It has ignored no avenue which has seemed a possible road to progress in this field, enlisting the aid of numerous agencies in its search. It is multidisciplinary in its approach, and in 1984 mounted a public exhibition in London on the theme of back pain.

CONCLUSION

The theme of this book is to present a profile of medical manipulation in the light of current knowledge. Inevitably, this will be modified as further evidence becomes available. Nevertheless, some matters are now clear, and these should be stated. The ideas and assertions purporting to present manipulation as a system of healing, with effects far beyond the relief of pain, have been shown to be invalid. For this reason, the 'mythology' of manipulation is currently at a low ebb. Further, we now have detailed physiological understanding of how these techniques work and of their relationships to several other forms of treatment, the efficacy of which depends upon the same mechanisms.

'In a general survey of the treatment of low back pain, it is pertinent to remember that with most of our patients we are uncertain of the true cause of their pain, and that present day methods of treatment suffer from this lack of knowledge'[140]. The fact is that, at present, 'in the great majority of cases we do not know the tissue or tissues from which back pain is originating or the cause of that pain. In the absence of an accurate diagnosis, controlled therapy is not possible. Therapeutic procedures, then, merely become empirical exercises'[4].

To quote Nachemson again, 'It is most beneficial to our patients and to ourselves to prescribe simple and inexpensive methods of treatment, using the known clinical, biological and mechanical factors to guide our advice'[140]. We contend that manipulation as portrayed in these pages fulfils these criteria. If the contraindications are strictly adhered to, it is a very safe form of treatment. The extreme paucity of material relating to postmanipulative complications supports this view. It is certainly inexpensive. The techniques described here are relatively simple and easy to deploy in general practice. In that unpredictable but substantial proportion of cases in which manipulation is helpful, this soon becomes apparent. Manipulation helps quickly or not at all.

In the light of this, we feel that the medical profession should look at these matters afresh. The existence of about 3500 lay manipulators in Britain indicates the popularity of this form of treatment with the public at large. At a time of therapeutic empiricism, all 'alternative' treatments, orthodox or unorthodox, should be considered. Given our present state of knowledge in this field, no one can reasonably say that any one form of treatment is markedly superior to another. None would deny, however, that manipulation has its successes. As diagnosis is most frequently uncertain, it seems unreasonable to withhold a form of therapy which, if employed as described, can do the patient no harm and may rapidly relieve the symptoms.

2
The Cervical Spine

FUNCTIONAL ANATOMY

The *cervical spine* is exceptionally mobile for the following reasons.

(1) the discal height relative to that of the vertebral body is 1 to 3, as against 1 to 6 in the thoracic spine and 1 to 3 in the lumbar spine[161],

(2) the smallness of the AP diameter of the vertebral body relative to this height,

(3) the sagittal facet angle of 45° permits movement in every direction, particularly flexion and extension,

(4) the anatomy of C1 and C2, atlas and axis.

The *atlas* has four functionally significant features:

(1) the posterior tubercle is small – permitting extension,

(2) the lateral processes extend a considerable distance, providing added leverage for rotation,

(3) as a consequence of this, however, the vertebral artery has to kink laterally to reach the foramen transversarium, and then back again to enter the occipital foramen,

(4) the vertebral foramen is large at the level of the atlas, the most mobile part of the spinal column, thus lessening the chances of cord compression.

The *axis* has two significant features:

(1) the dens, gripped to the anterior arch of the atlas by the transverse ligament, and with its own articular facets, clearly facilitates rotation, and

(2) the massive spine provides insertion for the long extensors of the neck.

The *joints*. There are six in the occipito-atlanto-axial complex, the facets for the dens, two between atlas and occiput and two between the atlas and axis. These are so shaped as to permit a marked AP rocking movement at the craniovertebral junction and substantial rotational movement at the atlantoaxial junction.

These joints are known in German, respectively, as the '*ja sager*' and the '*nein sager*'.

The joints of Luschka are formed between the elevated lateral edge of the upper surfaces of vertebral bodies 3–7 and the bevelled lower border of the vertebral body above. Their significance clinically is that they are very prone to osteophytosis which may involve neighbouring structures.

The zygoapophyseal joints

There are, of course, no zygoapophyseal joints between the atlanto-occipital and atlantoaxial levels. They are of great importance in mobility and, being weight-bearing, they are subject to osteophytosis[162]. The spinous processes are impalpable save for C7.

The *ligaments*. Most of the ligaments in the craniovertebral region are loose and weak, permitting considerable movements to take place at this level. There are two special ligaments: (1) the transverse to hold the dens to the arch of the atlas, thus protecting the cord, and (2) the alar ligaments from dens to occipital condyle to check rotation and, to a lesser extent, side-bending.

The sagittal diameter of the spinal canal at this point is 17 mm and that of the spinal cord, 10 mm[103]. Fielding, in 1971, showed that if the transverse ligaments were sectioned the arch was displaced forward by about 7 mm and by a further 3 mm if the alar ligaments were also sectioned[163]. The consequences of this will be considered later.

The muscles. The trapezius and splenius are extensors, the two recti and two obliques are primarily rotators. These muscles have a high innervation ratio in that the number of muscle fibres per motor neuron is small, being approximately three to five. In the sacrospin-alis muscles, the proportion is about 3000 muscle fibres per neuron. Therefore these smaller muscles, which have an innervation ratio as high as that of the external ocular muscles, are capable of very rapid and delicate movements.

Nerve supply

This is complexity itself, being far from segmental and being described by Stillwell in 1956[164] as being derived from a 'paravertebral plexus'. Wyke, in 1979, showed that the zygoapophyseal joint was innervated from *at least* three nerve roots, not only from its own segmentally related spinal nerve but also rostrally and caudally[165]. Kimmel, in 1961, showed that nerves from the upper three cervical segments supply the dura mater of the posterior cranial fossa, with the implications that may have in the production of headache[166]. An important fact is that the 5th cranial nerve nucleus descends in the spinal cord a considerable distance. It receives afferents from C1/C2/C3 dorsal nerve roots.

Anomalies

Bony asymmetry is very common in this area, with the implications that has for positional diagnosis. With regard to prefixation, i.e. the addition of C4, and postfixation, i.e. the addition of T2, to the brachial plexus both take in about 11% of cases of the population.

The movements of the cervical spine

Flexion/extension
The relevant degrees are as follows.

(1) At the atlanto-occipital joint, there is 20° of flexion, 30° of extension[161].

(2) The other cervical joints, in sequence, take part in this movement, giving a total in flexion of 20° ± 10°, extension 25° ± 10°[168].

Lateroflexion
The relevant degrees are as follows.

(1) The atlanto-occipital joint permits 15–20° restricted by the lateral ligaments.

(2) The atlas and axis permit only 5°. This movement is associated with a contralateral rotation.

(3)   The remainder contribute to give $45° \pm 10°$ each side[167], associated with ipsilateral rotation.

Rotation

Rotation of the head and neck is achieved by the synergistic action of ipsilateral splenius and contralateral sternomastoid. Atlas–axis rotate 30–35° to each side, approximately half the rotation of the cervical spine.

It must be remembered that all these figures are derived from radiological studies, and that they have limited clinical significance.

Movements of the cervical spine and manipulation

Manipulation of the upper cervical spine in flexion or extension affects particularly the atlantooccipital joint. Manipulation in rotation with contralateral lateroflexion affects the atlas–axis. Manipulation in rotation with ipsiflexion affects C2/C3. At the level of the middle or lower cervical spine lateroflexion, as a rule, should be done in the same direction as rotation (Maigne).

Some clinical consequences of upper cervical pathology

Rheumatoid arthritis

The neck is a site of predilection in this disease, and the transverse ligament is commonly involved. In 25% of cases flexion reveals a separation between the anterior surface of the dens and the posterior surface of the anterior arch of the atlas of 4 mm or more. The risk to the cord is self-evident. The principal danger to patients is in the hands of anaesthetists during induction of anaesthesia. Patients should therefore be sent to theatre wearing a collar to attract the attention of the anaesthetist[168]. Manipulation is contraindicated as it is in Grisel's syndrome (*see also* note in the section on Conventional Radiology of the cervical spine, below).

Arterial supply

The subclavian arteries give off the vertebral arteries which, passing through the foramina transversaria, unite above the atlas to form the basilar artery which, in turn, divides into right and left posterior cerebral arteries. Interference with these structures has long been known as being a cause of problems (thus Keuter, in 1970, in his article on 'vascular origin of cranial sensory disturbances caused by pathology of the lower cervical spine'[169]). The manipulative significance for these problems will be considered later. The blood supply of the cord is poor in the area of the cervical spine. This is why cervical myelopathy is the commonest neurological syndrome presenting after the age of 50 and is a contraindication for manipulation.

The course of the vertebral artery is such that it can give rise to potential fatalities due to thrombosis. Rotation and lateroflexion regularly stop the circulation in the vertebral artery on the opposite side. This has been proven by arteriography[91]. In the normal neck this is of no consequence, but in the presence of vascular disease it is a potential hazard.

SYMPTOMATOLOGY

Spinal problems are prone to have symptoms projected considerable distances from their origin.

The neck

The neck is a fruitful source of such syndromes.

1. Headache of cervical origin

That headache can arise from structures in the neck has been known in Britain since 1939, when Kellgren, by stimulating paravertebral structures in the upper cervical spine by injecting hypertonic saline, was able to produce referred pain experienced in the head[32]. In 1944, Campbell and Parsons injected irritant solutions into a variety of structures including capsules, fasciae and muscles and scratched the periosteum of upper cervical vertebrae with fine needles[170]. Of the 40 subjects, 20 were members of the hospital staff without previous head pain and 20 were patients who had been diagnosed as having head pain. These actions not only reproduced pains in the 'normal' subject very accurately felt by the real patients, but also produced a number of symptoms including giddiness, pallor, sweating, nausea and sometimes tinnitus. A notably strong resemblance between these symptoms and what they described as the 'post-traumatic head syndrome' was noted. It is remarkable that these two papers have had so little effect on medical thinking. In 1964, Trevor-Jones wrote a paper on the association between degenerative changes in the upper cervical spine and occipital headache[171]. In 1969, Dutton and Riley wrote that such changes could produce occipital headache not only from the upper cervical spine but with degenerative changes at any level between C2 and C7[172]. In 1974, Magora et al., in a series of 57 patients with headache, found a strong e.m.g. involvement of the semispinatous muscle in a high proportion of these cases[173]. Thus, there is now little doubt that cervical problems can cause headache.

The incidence of these problems is put by some authorities as being one in three. Therefore, routine analysis of any headache must involve examination of the cervical spine. The topography of these conditions is 75% supraorbital, 20% occipital, 5% radiating to the ear, and in up to 5% pain is radiated from occiput to vertex (Arnold's neuralgia)[91].

In the absence of contraindications and in the presence of positive signs, manipulation is the treatment of choice. Results are excellent in eight cases out of ten. The unsuccessful involve either a psychological component or a degree of severity suggesting the use of injections.

2. Migraine

Frykholm in 1971 wrote, 'In my experience cervical migraine is the type of headache most frequently seen in general practice and also the type most frequently misinterpreted. It is usually erroneously diagnosed as classic migraine, tension headache, vascular headache, hypertensive encephalopathy or post-traumatic encephalopathy. Such patients have usually received inadequate treatment and have often become neurotic and drug-dependent'[33].

Friedman, in 1975, claimed that classic migraine occurred in about 10% of patients diagnosed as having migraine[174]. Sheldon, in 1967, produced the results of a survey of 109 patients who had been admitted to hospital over 15 years for headache and had been diagnosed as having migraine[175]. He found that as many as 67 of them had what he described as the cervico-occipital syndrome. It is clear from this material that this diagnosis is frequently made in error for what are in fact headaches of cervical origin.

True migraine is a syndrome of recurrent unilateral headaches associated with pallor, nausea and photophobia and preceded by prodromal symptoms such as fortification spectra. Manipulation has no part to play in the treatment of this condition. However, cervical spinal problems can produce recurrent unilateral headaches which are understandably misdiagnosed as migraine. Moreover, true migraine can coexist with a spinal condition. If, therefore, examination reveals positive local signs, treatment in the former group will be curative in the great majority of cases, and it will often modify the situation for the better in the latter.

3. ENT symptoms of cervical origin

Mention has already been made of the work of Campbell and Parsons who showed, *inter alia*, a variety of bizarre ENT symptoms could be produced from cervical structures[170]. In 1959, Cope and Ryan established a connection between some cervical disorders and vertigo[176]. In 1969, Toglia, Rosenberg and Ronis studied 72 patients who had suffered whiplash injury to the neck[177]. They examined them with tests of vestibular function, audiometry and electronystamography and found positive correlation in more than two thirds of cases. Kosoy and Glassman, in 1974, in patients who had suffered cervical spinal trauma and who presented with bizarre symptoms, found, on objective ENT evaluation, objective abnormalities in 50% of cases[178]. In 1974, Dionne wrote a paper entitled 'Neck torsion nystagmus'[179]. As can be seen, the connection between cervical spinal problems and these often bizarre symptoms is far from fanciful. Nevertheless, this fact is not widely appreciated, and these patients are frequently still regarded with suspicion.

In practice, these patients almost invariably have been given a clean bill of health. Diagnosis is by routine examination of the neck. Treatment, in the absence of contraindications and in the presence of positive signs, is manipulation.

However, if any symptoms are present suggesting basilar artery involvement, manipulation is absolutely contraindicated, as is assessment of global cervical movement.

4. Post-traumatic headache

The connection between headache and trauma has already been touched upon. In 1967, Jackson analysed a series of 5500 cases of cervical spinal disorders[180]. Of these, 85% had been as a result of trauma and headache was one of the most frequent complaints voiced. Roca, in 1972, reported a series of 15 patients with marked ocular disturbances following whiplash injury[181].

5. Torticollis

This condition can be defined as a postural deformity with the head in flexion and side flexion away from the painful side. This description of a position, however, scarcely constitutes a pathological diagnosis which is presumably multifactorial. The onset of this syndrome is variable. However, as a point of interest, Spisak, in 1972, noted that in a series of 103 cases, 80% could not localize their pain[182]. If mild, this condition is suitable for treatment by manipulation in the pain-free direction (Maigne[91]). If not, it responds well to injections as described later in this chapter, in the section on Injections. Mehta, in 1973, wrote that this condition is frequently aided by a nerve-block at the level C2/C3[145].

Brachial and thoracic radiation

All forelimb pain demands cervical assessment. Arm pain may either occupy known nerve root topography or not.

Jackson in 1966 wrote, 'pain in or about the shoulder joint, from irritation of cervical nerve roots, may give rise to reflex sympathetic dystrophy with resulting changes in capsular tendons. Similar changes may occur at elbow, wrist and fingers'[180].

Cervical neurology

C5   Shoulder pain extending to the elbow; muscle weakness may occur in deltoid, infraspinatus, biceps

C6   Pain may involve the anterolateral border of the shoulder and the lateral border of the arm to the thumb; the biceps and radiostyloid reflexes may be involved; weakness may involve the biceps, supraspinatus muscles and those of the thenar eminence

C7   Posterior surface of shoulder and arm to index and third finger;

the triceps reflex may be involved; muscle weakness may involve the triceps and extensors of the hand and fingers

C8 Pain is felt at the medial border of the arm and wrist and in the fourth and fifth fingers; power involves the extensors of the thumb

In practice, reflex changes are rare, and muscle weakness considerably more so. In all cases of arm pain other pathologies must be excluded, e.g. Pancoast's syndrome, other neoplasms and syringomyelia. In all cases of shoulder pain the neck, again, must be assessed.

Acroparaesthesiae

These are symptoms of numbness, tingling and pins and needles. They must be classified in four groups:

(1) global acroparaesthesiae – involving the whole hand and usually nocturnal,

(2) radicular acroparaesthesiae (*see above*),

(3) carpal tunnel syndrome, and

(4) acroparaesthesiae of neurological origin (syringomyelia).

The carpal tunnel syndrome is suspected:

(a) if symptoms occur in the territory of the median nerve, i.e. the first three fingers and half of the fourth,

(b) if flexion of the wrist or pressure over the canal – maintained for a minute – will reproduce symptoms,

(c) if relief can be obtained by injecting local steroid or by surgery,

(d) if there is a delay of nerve conduction time assessed by e.m.g.

In the presence of cervical signs, manipulation of groups (a) and (b) is not only legitimate but logical. In group (c) its function is less clear but, used in conjunction with other treatments, it is frequently effective. 'It is as if the irritation of the cervical root was responsible for a state of congestion or oedema at the level of the carpal tunnel' (Maigne[91]).

Tennis elbow

Thirty per cent of cases are purely cervical in origin, 30% have a cervical and a local component, and the remainder have local signs, in the absence of cervical signs. In the first group treatment is cervical, in the second it is cervical and local, and in the remainder of cases it is local.

Of particular interest in this connection is a paper by Gunn and Millbrandt in 1976 regarding 50 patients who had failed to respond to 4 weeks of conservative local treatment[183]. These authors then directed treatment to the patients' necks (but not manipulation). They used mobilization, cervical traction, isometric exercises and heat or ultrasound. Forty-seven patients responded and, of these, 44 who were re-assessed at 3 months and 6 months remained symptom-free.

Golfer's elbow

As in tennis elbow, a cervical origin must always be sought.

Thoracic radiation

The great majority of cases of thoracic pain are cervical rather than thoracic in origin. Typically they present with interscapular pain and the interscapular point (*see above*). Cloward has proved that stimulation of the anterolateral part of the discs at the level of C4, C5, C6 and C7 reproduces interscapular pain[34]. Thus, in any case of thoracic pain, the cervical spine must be examined and, if appropriate, treated.

It must be remembered that pain from the lower cervical spine can be referred anteriorly (*see* the 'bell-push' sign of Maigne, illustrated in Chapter 7).

EXAMINATION

Posture

As in other regions of the spine, postural abnormalities should be sought and recorded.

Global movements

In the young adult

(1) normal flexion should permit the chin to touch the sternum,

(2) normal extension should permit vertical vision,

(3) in lateroflexion, the ear should touch the shoulder,

(4) in rotation, the chin should touch the acromioclavicular joint.

The measurement of these movements is not diagnostic, but provides a means of recording clinical response to treatment.

Neurology

Resisted movements may demonstrate relative weakness suggesting involvement of nerve roots at the levels indicated:

rotation of neck	C5/C6
shrugging of shoulders	C2/C3/C4
abduction and lateral rotation of shoulder	C5
flexion at elbow	C5/C6
extension at wrist	C6
extension at elbow	C7
flexion at wrist	C7
ulnar deviation at wrist	C8
extension and abduction of thumb	C8
proximation of 4th and 5th fingers	T1

While an essential part of the examination, it may be observed that in practice, positive signs are rare.

Tendon reflexes

Asymmetry of tendon reflexes may demonstrate involvement of nerve roots at the levels indicated:

biceps	C5/C6
supinator	C5/C6
triceps	C7

Local examination

Patient standing or sitting
Palpatory tests are made
    (1) skin drag and
    (2) skin rolling.

Patient supine

Palpation
Palpate paravertebral musculature, to observe differences in muscle tone on the two sides.

Pressure
(1)   Springing (pressure over the spinous processes)
(2)   Lateral pressure – impossible for anatomical reasons, save at C7

Apophyseal signs
This is a tenderness sought for at one finger's breadth paramedially and corresponds anatomically to a posterior articular joint, probably tender periarticular tissues and, at this level, possibly the posterior branch of a spinal nerve. This sign is of capital importance, as effective treatment by injection may produce dramatically beneficial results.

The anterior 'bellpush' test (Maigne) should be used not only because it may reveal pain referred from the cervical to the thoracic area, but also because it emphasizes the importance of anterior palpation. Similar signs are the eyebrow and jaw tests of Maigne, all of which are illustrated in Chapter 7.

CONVENTIONAL RADIOLOGY

The basic considerations have been given in the section on Conventional Radiology in Chapter 1. In the cervical spine degenerative changes are common. Olsson, in 1942, showed that over the age of 60, incidence of arthrosis in the atlanto-dental joint was 88%[184]. Trevor-Jones, in 1964, demonstrated that osteophytic change is common, sometimes unilaterally, at the C2/C3 zygoapophyseal Joint[171]. Finneson, in 1969, showed that these degenerative changes could not only compress the vertebral artery, but sometimes artery and nerve together[185]. Keuter, in 1970, demonstrated that vascular pathology in the cervical spine could project signs and symptoms considerable distances[169]. Thus, one patient had problems with disturbances of sensation in the left hemicranial region, headaches and vertigo, and also disturbances of sensation in the C6/C7/C8 territory of the left arm. Degenerative changes were found to coexist radiologically. Phillips, in 1975, found that there was no close correlation between radiological changes and clinical features, as has been demonstrated elsewhere in the spine[186] (*see* Chapter 3, Conventional Radiology section). Thus, von Torklus, in 1972, wrote, 'It has to be kept in mind that there is no strict inter-dependence between clinical symptoms and radiological pathology in the cranio-vertebral region'[187].

Radiology has an important part to play in the diagnosis of Grisel's syndrome since it is the only objective way of demonstrating cervical hypermobility. In 1970, Gutmann was able to demonstrate this in a group of affected children[66]. As the detection on palpation of segmental hyper- and hypomobility has been used to diagnose spinal lesions and monitor their treatment, so has conventional radiology. In fact, radiological hyper- and hypomobility and their responses to manipulative treatment have never been conclusively demonstrated. The fact that Swezey and Silverman, in 1971, showed that the overriding of zygoapophyseal joints of 3 mm in the middle of the cervical spine and 3·5 mm at the level of S/5 and S/1 were not detectable on routine X-rays indicates the difficulty of such endeavours[188].

With regard to inflammatory arthritides, Sharp and Purser in 1961, in a paper on spontaneous atlantoaxial dislocation in ankylosing spondylitis and rheumatoid arthritis, showed that the cervical spine was involved in 40% of cases of rheumatoid arthritis[189]. The incidence of atlantoaxial displacement has been studied by Mathews in 1969[190] and Conlon *et al.*[191] in 1966, and is usually agreed as being around 25% taking as the criterion the separation of the odontoid peg from the posterior surface of the anterior arch of the atlas by 4 mm or more. Nor is rheumatoid arthritis confined to the atlantoaxial region as a fatal dislocation at the level of C4/C5 has been reported by Whaley and Dick in 1968[192]. Moreover, it has also been demonstrated that the severity of radiological changes does not correlate with the severity of clinical features. Therefore, manipulation of the rheumatoid neck is clearly strongly contra-indicated (*see* Chapter 1, section on Indications, Contraindications and Dangers).

INJECTIONS

1.   Injection of 'trigger' areas

This is frequently used in the cervical area, particularly of the inter-vertebral ligaments between the transverse processes of C4–C6. Wilkinson observes that the injection of tender areas in cervical spondylosis gives relief of pain and spasm and improves cervical movements[193]. Maigne described tender and thickened eyebrow tissues related to upper cervical joint problems[56]. These could be eradicated by either local manipulation or injection of the upper cervical spine. Materials used vary. We commonly use 2 ml of local anaesthetic and 2 ml of steroid.

2.   Nerve block

The commonest use of this technique in the cervical area is for headaches caused by the greater occipital nerve (C2) in Arnold's neuralgia. The surface marking is either tenderness or reproduction of pain on palpation (rare) one-finger's breadth medial to the mastoid process.

3.   Attachment tissues

The myofascial attachments of trapezius, sternomastoid and splenius capitis to the occiput are often found to be tender on palpation between mastoid process and the midline. Infiltration with the above materials is frequently helpful. It will be noted that there is overlap here between this instance and the injection of C2. Wide infiltration in both cases is desirable.

4.   Periarticular injection around apophyseal joints

This is widely used in the cervical area and is becoming more so. The clinical indications are acute torticollis, or a painful neck with tenderness over the apophyseal joints. These cases may be impossible to manipulate because of the severity of symptoms, or technically difficult because of the apprehension of the patient, with resultant failure to relax.

The surface marking
This is a tenderness one finger's breadth from the midline. It is common to feel a tender mass thought to be periarticular tissues and muscles in spasm. This 'mass' led to the illusion held originally by lay osteopaths that a 'bone was out of place'.

Technique
The patient should be seated, and told to look up and to hold still. This will ensure the superimposition of the laminae. A $1\frac{1}{2}$-inch (38 mm) disposable needle is used with a 5 ml solution of local anaesthetic and steroid. The needle is inserted until bone is struck, the plunger is withdrawn to ensure a blood vessel is not involved. Sometimes, synovial fluid from the facet joint is obtained. So much the better. 2 ml is given directly and then the needle angled half an inch (13 mm) upward and half an inch downward and half the residue of the fluid is given at each site. Because of the eccentric course of the vertebral artery between C2 and the foramen magnum this can be injected with serious and even fatal consequences. Therefore, injection above the level of C2 is absolutely contraindicated for the beginner. Even the experienced practitioner must exercise the greatest care to ensure that blood vessels are not involved.

An alternative technique has the patient prone, resting his chin on the couch so as to superimpose the laminae. To further reduce the risk of entering the spinal canal, the needle is very nearly withdrawn after the first injection, then slid with the skin cranially to the level immediately above, the needle once more being directed vertically until it meets bone, the process being repeated for the third part of the injection by sliding the needle point and skin caudally to the level below the original injection.

3
The Thoracic Spine

FUNCTIONAL ANATOMY

This is the least mobile segment of the spinal column

(1) because of attachments of the rib cage

(2) because the discs are thin, comprising only one seventh of the height of the vertebral bodies.

Vertebral bodies

Twelve in number, these are short, diminishing in size from T1 to T3 then increasing to T12 which shares the same general mass and shape as the lumbar vertebrae.

Ligaments

These are the same as elsewhere in the spinal column, anterior and posterior longitudinal ligaments, inter- and supraspinous ligaments, intertransverse ligaments and the ligamentum flavum. Thicker than in the cervical spine, these are less dense than in the lumbar spine.

Joints

Costovertebral
The head of the rib is inserted into a concavity formed by adjacent vertebral bodies and the disc between. It is secured by a fibrous capsule and the fan-shaped radiate ligament.

Costotransverse
The typical rib, halfway between head and angle, articulates with the front of the transverse process of the numerically corresponding

vertebra. It has a capsule and three costotransverse ligaments and is important in restricting thoracic movement.

Zygoapophyseal joints
These are practically vertical from the lateral point of view and, therefore, restrict rotation.

Thoraco-lumbar joint
At a variable level (T10/T11, T11/T12, T12/L1) the apophyseal joints change from thoracic to lumbar in type. This means that the upper joints are thoracic, the lower being lumbar in type.

Blood vessels
These form extraordinarily complicated anastomoses. From T4 to T9 the spinal canal is at its narrowest and the blood supply to the cord is at its poorest. Therefore, any patient who has low back symptoms and thoracic spinal problems is a potential manipulative hazard.

Nerve supply
The nerve supply, like the vasculature, is extremely complex and interrelated. The sinu-vertebral nerve may wander up and down four or five segments before terminating. The disproportion between cord and column length means the upper thoracic roots have to travel down 3 cm to reach the foraminal exits, while at the thoracolumbar junction 7 cm. Clinically, T12 supplies the buttock, and hence low back pain may be thoracic in origin.

Anomalies
Thoracic spinous processes are frequently asymmetrical by up to 5 mm. Therefore, 'positional' diagnosis is particularly misleading in this region. Also the obliquity of the spinous processes may lead to difficulty in the identification of the precise anatomical level in question.

SYMPTOMATOLOGY

It is commonly held by clinicians, ourselves included, that in this area static work posture is of particular importance. Back pain associated with typing or dressmaking is common in this region. To prove that this is the case is, however, unfortunately exceptionally difficult. Thus a number of workers, including Partridge and Anderson, in 1969[194], and Magora, in 1974[195], found a positive correlation between back symptomatology where subjects sat for long periods of time. Braun, in 1969[196], and Svensson and Andersson, in 1983[197], have not confirmed this correlation. The chief difficulty, or virtual impossibility, is that of isolating the various factors that may be involved. These are not only physical. Aaras, in 1982, introduced ergonomic changes in a Norwegian factory which reduced sick leave due to back pain[198]. However, during this time, there was also a change in the pay system that happened to be popular with the workforce and this may have had an influence on reduction of sick leave due to these problems. 'There is, nevertheless', Aaras concluded, 'a clear indication that the ergonomic annotations had a positive influence on the health of the workers.'

It has been emphasized elsewhere that pain is commonly radiated into the thoracic area from the cervical spine[91], classically in the work of Frykholm[199] and Cloward[34]. It is also emphasized elsewhere that pain from the thoracolumbar region is commonly radiated to the buttock and the low back. This led Maigne to claim that 60% of low back pain either is solely of thoracolumbar origin or occurs in association with lumbosacral problems.

It is of great clinical importance to consider pain of thoracic vertebral origin perceived as originating in chest or abdomen. As long ago as 1955, Prinzmetal and Massumi noted that cardiac patients may also have musculoskeletal problems of the chest wall[200]. They evolved a point system for differentiating between these two forms of chest pain. They wrote, 'It is entirely possible that somatic anterior chest wall pain is pathologically analogous to the shoulder hand syndrome'. Other authors, e.g. Allison in 1950[201] and Edwards in 1955[202], quoted many cases in which pain felt in the chest wall was musculoskeletal in origin and had nothing whatsoever to do with cardiac problems. Professor Fossgreen, observing admissions to Aarhuis Hospital in Denmark over a period of 2 years for chest pain, found that in 20% of cases the pain was musculoskeletal[203]. Grant and Keegan, in 1968, have described cases where people have chest pain of musculoskeletal origin, this being demonstrated by it being brought on by movements of the thoracic spine, such as twisting, bending or turning in bed[204].

Marinacci and Courville, in 1962, presented a series of cases that had been operated upon due to an error of diagnosis, the pain in fact being spinal in origin[205]. One such patient had been operated on no fewer than three times. 'The resultant abdominal manifestations can usually be traced to stem from irritation of one or more thoracic spinal roots ... in this group of syndromes we are concerned with the entire abdominal wall supplied by the sensory and motor roots from about T6 down to L1 level.' In 1977, Ashby studied 73 patients who he found to have abdominal pain of spinal origin and which he treated with nerve blocks[206]. 'Spinal root or referred pain often arise synchronously and in the same segments as visceral abnormalities either because of summation or through visceroparietal reflexes. The possibility of vertebral problems and the need for examination, including local examination, is therefore essential. An acute abdomen may be simulated by aching from skeletal structures in febrile illness'. Therefore, it can be seen that this problem is quite common. It is far from sufficiently appreciated clinically at the present time. The symptoms are sometimes so marked that the vertebral cause of the problem is obscured.

It is therefore clear that local examination is of great importance in cases of apparent visceral disorder and that, *in this context a purely conventional clinical examination is inadequate.*

EXAMINATION

Posture

As in other regions of the spine, postural abnormalities should be sought and recorded.

Global movements

For the sake of convenience, these are divided into flexion, extension, side-bending and rotation. In each case, what is sought is pain on movement, with or without apparent restriction of that particular movement. It must be remembered that these movements are of significance in the monitoring of the results of therapy rather than in making a specific diagnosis.

Neurological examination

There is no conventional neurological examination specifically applicable to the thoracic spine.

Local examination

1. Palpatory

Tests are

(1)   skin drag,
(2)   skin rolling and
(3)   paravertebral muscle palpation.

2. Pressure

(1)   springing of the spinous processes
(2)   lateral pressure to spinous processes
(3)   pressure over the apophyseal joints.

3. Anterior referral

Given that symptoms and signs can be referred considerable distances from the point of their vertebral origin, it is necessary to examine the whole spine whatever the problem presenting. No one section can be examined in isolation.

An example of this is the cervical *point sonnette* (the cervical bell-push sign) of Maigne. The point of anterior tenderness felt over the anterolateral part of the cervical spine is a point not only of local tenderness but which will frequently, on being pressed, radiate pain down into the thorax. Attention should be directed to the level of the cervical spine at which this sign is elicited. This also emphasizes the point that since pain and tenderness can be referred anteriorly, examination is not complete without careful anterior palpation. This is particularly important with regard to the thoracic spine where pain may be referred to the anterior chest wall or to the abdomen, simulating visceral disease.

A particular point of clinical interest is the existence of the 'interscapular point'[91]. In many cases, patients will complain of pain between the shoulder blades, and pressure one finger's breadth lateral to the spinous process will elicit a tender spot, reproducing the initial symptoms. The site to be treated, however, is considerably higher. This is because the posterior branches of the spinal nerves in the thoracic spine descend three to four levels before cutaneous inner-vation occurs. Thus dealing with an involved posterior branch, clinical signs may be found at two levels. The pressure test will be positive where the branch emerges spinally and the interscapular point will be found several levels lower down.

CONVENTIONAL RADIOLOGY

General radiological considerations have been set out in Chapter 1, in the section on Conventional Radiology. With regard to the thor-acic spine, so-called degenerative changes are as common here as they are elsewhere in the vertebral column. Nathan, in a study in 1964, found that in a series of 346 spines, he first detected such changes between the ages of 20 and 30, these changes rapidly increas-ing to a maximum between the ages of 40 and 50[207]. They were commonest at the upper and lower ends of the thoracic spine.

Changes indicating thoracic spondylosis are very common indeed. Nathan and Schwarz, in 1962[208], contended that osteophytes tended to be formed on the anterior and right lateral aspect of the vertebral bodies. They also showed that these changes, presumably because of the concavity of this region, were more marked anteriorly. Scheuermann's disease was first described by this Swiss radiologist in 1920[209]. Features are kyphosis, wedging of vertebral bodies anteriorly, narrow disc spaces and the presence of Schmorl's nodes. Although these changes are most marked in the thoracic spine, they are also common in both cervical and lumbar spines[210]. It is of clinical interest that Stoddard has shown that although the incidence overall is 13% in the population, it can be demonstrated in 49% of people with low back pain. Scott showed, in 1974, that vertebral collapse due to osteoporosis was most commonly to be found in the thoracic or upper lumbar region of the spine[212].

INJECTIONS

Injections in the thoracic region are of great value and may be a potent means of reducing pain.

Trigger points

These have been described as tender areas in muscles and soft tissues associated with palpable nodules. Injection of these nodules with local anaesthetic often results in abolition of pain, an effect which frequently outlasts the known duration of efficacy of the drug employed. Resolution of pain is commonly accompanied by disappearance of the nodules[148].

Peripheral nerve block

This may be attempted in 'encircling' pain relating to a particular segment. Injection may be made at the point where the posterior branch curls round to supply the apophyseal joint capsule, or where it is accessible at the inferior aspect of the costotransverse joint. The latter requires considerable care in avoiding penetration of the subjacent pleura. Local anaesthetic and steroid mixtures are used. These injections should not be attempted in general practice, as they are difficult and potentially dangerous.

Rib fractures

Local anaesthetic and steroid mixtures are extremely helpful in rib fractures, the aim being to deaden pain by placing the injection in the vicinity of the periosteum, as near to the fracture site as possible. The same technique is applicable to costochondral strain or displacement, also requiring care in avoiding pleural puncture.

Apophyseal joints

These may be found approximately one finger's breadth from the midline and may be tender. Introduction of local anaesthetic into the joint is not necessary, and in purely clinical practice is not likely to be achieved. However, this is of no consequence, as infiltration adjacent to the posterior capsule is often sufficient to produce the desired effect with the mixture described.

Sclerosants

There are those who use sclerosants in the thoracic spine, but they remain in a minority at present.

The omission of costotransverse and costovertebral injections from this discussion is deliberate, because of the rarity of these problems and the dangers of pueumothorax such techniques can involve.

4
The Lumbar Spine

FUNCTIONAL ANATOMY

Vertebral bodies

These are five in number, the region having an anterior convexity, which is scarcely surprising in view of the stresses put upon it.

Apophyseal joints

These are true synovial joints, virtually anteroposterior in plane. Thus flexion and extension are free (30° flexion and 20° extension). Lateroflexion (20°–30°) and rotation (10°) are relatively limited. In particular they restrict AP glide at the intervertebral joints. The intervertebral discs account for one third of the height of the lumbar spine in the healthy young adult. Their component parts are described individually, but together they form the basis of the mobile segment, taking the stresses of weight bearing and permitting a strictly limited mobility of the whole[213].

(1) *The annulus fibrosus* is a fibrocartilaginous ring which has no nerve supply. However, the outer fibres of its posterior surface are closely associated with the posterior longitudinal ligament which has, of course, a lavish nociceptor system. For this reason events at this site can cause pain. It is constructed of layers of fibroelastic tissue, the fibres running obliquely between the margins of the vertebral bodies above and below, in alternate directions, the attachments being very strong. It encloses the nucleus pulposus.

(2) *The nucleus pulposus* comprises about 40% of the intervertebral disc and is a readily deformable, though non-compressible, semi-fluid gel. Contained within the annulus fibrosus, it is separated

from the vertebral bodies above and below by the hyaline cartilage plates.

(3) *The hyaline cartilage plate* is the growth centre for much of the
vertebral body, helps to anchor the fibres of the annulus fibrosus peripherally, and transmits the compression force between
vertebral bodies through the nucleus pulposus, at the same time
separating the nucleus from the vascular spongiosa of the vertebral bodies.

Thus the intervertebral disc is in effect a self-contained, semihy-
draulic shock-absorber system, permitting movement in shear, in
rotation, in tilt and (by distending the annulus fibrosus) in compression. Under load it changes shape, the force applied between vertebral bodies being transmitted equally in all directions by the nucleus
pulposus. The effect of this hydraulic pressure is to distort the annulus fibrosus asymmetrically, depending upon its local strength and
the pre-stressing of its fibres by positional factors.

The posterior portion of the annulus fibrosus is a site of potential
weakness because:

(1) the fibres are thin posteriorly,

(2) gravitational pressure is applied more heavily posteriorly[31],

(3) the posterior longitudinal ligament is thinner over the disc than
it is over the vertebral body and

(4) in flexion, and under load of a lifting strain, the nucleus pulposus is pressed posteriorly against the overstretched posterior
fibres of the annulus fibrosus.

Ligaments

These are generally stronger and thicker than elsewhere. The ilio-
lumbar ligaments attach the 5th spinous and transverse processes to
the posterior iliac crest.

Heylings, in 1978, has shown that the lumbosacral ligament, contrary to popular belief, does not exist[214]. Below the spinous process
of L5, the structures present are fibres of decussating lumbar fascia.
The density of nociceptive innervation in ligaments is greatest in the
posterior longitudinal ligament, less in the sacroiliac and other longitudinal ligaments and least in the ligamentum flavum.

Blood vessels

These form an extremely complex system of arterial and venous anastomoses.

Nerves

The nerves form a system as complex and intricate as that of the blood vessels.

Because the spinal cord ends at the level of L1, the lower roots have a variable but lengthy journey within the canal before they emerge at their respective intervertebral foramina. They are intimately related to the posterior aspects of the discs, with the possibility this offers for root involvement in disc abnormalities or disease. Thus, a recurrent branch of L2 may descend to the L5 level and, therefore, can be a misleading source of back pain[215].

Anomalies

Structural abnormalities (spina bifida, sacralization of L5) are common. They are commonly found in pain-free subjects (*see* Epstein in 1969 in a review of spinal studies of patients admitted to hospital with problems other than back pain). This was also shown by La Rocca and Macnab in 1969 on 3000 pre-employment X-rays taken over 2 years[217].

Degenerative changes

The combination of congenital or acquired distortion of the spinal canal, resulting in the unpredictable diminution of its cross-sectional area, due to spondylosis and spondylolisthesis, is a common occurrence and provides structural abnormalities (particularly in the elderly) which may or may not produce symptoms. Spondylosis may also affect the root canals, in addition to the spinal canal.

Spinal stenosis is now attracting far more attention than has previously been the case. 'It is much more common than hitherto appreciated'[218]. Weinstein, in 1979, wrote that material relating to stenosis had either failed to be published or, if published, had been ignored[219].

Physiology

Most of the structures mentioned can and do serve as sources of pain.

Clinical consequences of lumbar anatomy

(1) Because of the thickness of muscle and other tissues, palpation is of less help here than in the neck.

(2) Because of the variety of tissues and structures which may be involved in producing pain, and the complexity of innervation, the site and radiation of pain as a symptom is of relatively little diagnostic help.

A CLASSIFICATION OF LOW BACK PAIN

The importance of the activities of daily living, posture and prophylaxis have been emphasized in Chapter 1, in the section on Posture and Prophylaxis. In view of the vagaries of referred pain and referred tenderness, we feel that it would be of help to offer a classification of low back pain. This is based on the chapter, 'The neurology of low back pain', by Professor B. Wyke, in the 1980 edition of Jayson's *The Lumbar Spine and Back Pain*[215]. For our purpose, low back pain is defined as pain experienced in the lumbosacral region. The four basic groups are primary backache, secondary backache, referred backache and psychosomatic backache.

Primary backache

This is defined as low back pain resulting from direct mechanical or chemical irritation of the nociceptor nerve endings embedded in the various lumbosacral tissues.

Cutaneous pain
This category presents little diagnostic difficulty and will therefore not be discussed.

Pain originating in muscles and fascia

A common cause of back pain is the irritation of nociceptors situated in the muscle masses of the lower back, and their fascial sheaths and intramuscular septa, and those in the tendons that attach them to the vertebral column and pelvis. Such irritation is usually caused by mechanical trauma, reflex spasm or muscle fatigue. Inflammatory causes are much rarer.

Trauma

This may lead to tearing of some of the tendinous attachments of muscles to bone or periosteum, or to the rupture of muscle fibres and tearing of their fascial sheaths. The initial pain is due to the factors already detailed, while prolonged, subsequent pain is due to irritation of the same nerve endings as a result of the chemical changes that occur in the interstitial fluid of the damaged tissues.

Muscle spasm

When excessive motor activity is maintained for prolonged periods in any muscle, pain may develop, and the muscle may also become tender. This occurs because of irritation of unmyelinated nerve fibres, distributed in the adventitial sheaths of the intramuscular blood vessels, due to chemical changes that develop in the interstitial fluid of the muscles, in turn resulting from the abnormal metabolic activity of the hyperactive muscle fibres. This may arise from abnormal activity of the receptors located in the joints of the vertebral column because of postural abnormalities or degenerative changes in the vertebral column (i.e. degenerative disc disease or osteoarthrosis). It may also result from irritative lesions involving segmentally related viscera, especially the genitourinary system. It will be noted how great is the variety of possible causes and sources of reflex muscle spasm.

Muscle fatigue

Muscles subjected to prolonged work become fatigued and both painful and tender. Particularly is this so with regard to the back muscles when they are subjected to postural abnormalities over a period of time, or as a result of the demands of occupation or athletic activity. The cause is not fully understood, but it does depend upon inadequate muscle blood flow and may arise from biochemical changes in the muscles similar to that of reflex muscle spasm. Electromyographic appearances presented by fatigued muscles differ, however, from those in muscles in spasm. It should be noted that backache associated with postural, occupational fatigue is not necessarily derived from the nociceptor systems in the back muscles, since it may well come from mechanical irritation of nerve endings in the lumbar spinal ligaments or in the capsules of the apophyseal joints or the sacro-iliac joints. It is also of clinical interest to note that it can be relieved by measures promoting blood flow, such as massage and heat.

Inflammation
Fibrositis has never been histologically demonstrated, therefore there is no evidence that it exists. Myositis, being a non-suppurative inflammation of muscles, is most commonly seen in clinical practice in association with viral diseases such as influenza. However, inflammatory causes of back pain are much less common than muscular fatigue, spasm or trauma.

Articular and ligamentous pain
The only common cause of primary back pain, other than myofascial pain, lies in irritation of nociceptor systems distributed in the fibrous capsules of the lumbar apophyseal and sacro-iliac joints and throughout the ligaments related to the vertebral column.

Articular pain
Abnormal mechanical stresses can arise from poor posture, from the development of weakness or atrophy of back muscles as a result of ageing or from the reduction of vertical height of the lumbar spine (for example in osteoporosis, vertebral body collapse, or as a result of intervertebral disc generation). Articular pain may also arise from manipulation under general anaesthesia or from putting women into the Trendelenburg position (for example), by means of placing unacceptable strains upon lumbar apophyseal capsules. Inflammatory changes involving these fibrous capsules are most commonly seronegative and seropositive arthritides. In this latter case, the pain is determined exclusively by the inflammatory involvement of the capsules, since the articular cartilages, intra-articular menisci and synovial tissue contain no nerve endings of any kind. It follows that

radiological changes, however marked, have no direct correlation with the severity of the backache.

Ligamentous pain

Irritation of the receptor systems in ligaments is associated with irritation of nerve endings located in the joint capsules. It has been thought that static postural support for the lower spine in the erect, sitting and fully-flexed positions of the body is provided by the passive, elastic tension of the ligaments and aponeuroses, rather than by muscular activity. Whether this is true is not clear, but all these structures are richly innervated with nociceptive nerve endings, and it is clear that backache arising from postural abnormalities of the vertebral column can be readily provoked, as it can by lifting strains. A substantial proportion of the so-called fatigue backache encountered in everyday life probably results from this ligamentous source in the first place, which may be reinforced by irritation of nociceptive systems in the back muscles and joint capsules. Disc protrusion can cause direct mechanical irritation of the nerve endings in the posterior longitudinous ligament and in the fibrous and adipose tissue that binds it to the annulus fibrosus, or may be produced by central posterior protrusion of the nucleus pulposus.

Bony pain

This may be caused either by irritation of the perivascular system distributed throughout the cancellous bone of the vertebral bodies and arches, and of the sacrum, or of lesions involving the enclosing periosteum. The causes of such problems are trauma to the lower back, especially in the case of crush fractures of the lumbar vertebral bodies, the collapse of vertebral bodies as a result of osteomalacia or osteoporosis, or secondary neoplasm, derived in particular from the prostate, uterus, breast, colon, bladder and thyroid.

Vascular pain

This is more common than is frequently supposed, arising from mechanical irritation of the nerve endings in the walls of the vertebral venous plexus, as a result of excessive distension of these vessels by the development of abnormally high venous pressures. The vertebral venous system is in direct communication with veins in the chest, abdomen and pelvis, and therefore elevation of pressure in these cavities is transmitted freely to, and provokes distension of, the vertebral veins. Such elevation of venous pressure may be high in acts of lifting or supporting heavy weights, as the abdominal and thoracic muscles then contract after deep inspiration against a closed glottis. The same mechanism is at play in sneezing, coughing and vomiting.

Dural pain

While the dural tube has little or no nociceptive innervation on its posterior surface, it is densely supplied on its anterior surface and in the dural sleeves extending into the intervertebral foramina. Pressure from a bulging or prolapsed intervertebral disc onto these structures produces pain. This may be compounded by the presence of osteophytes, in spinal stenosis and in spondylolisthesis.

Summary

It is clear from the above that nociceptive receptor systems are present in many lumbosacral tissues. It is also evident that the causative factors in low back pain are numerous, while the mechanisms of pain production are identical, so that pain may arise from several tissues simultaneously. In addition to this, stimulation of any of these systems, alone or in concert, can cause paravertebral muscle spasm which in itself may be painful. It is evident, as has been shown above, that in many instances, in a given episode of back pain, several different tissues may be involved at the same time. It is also clear that the attempt to identify the tissue or tissues from which such pain may be arising is indeed a difficult enterprise.

Secondary backache

This may be defined as pain experienced in the lumbosacral region as a result of disturbance of function of the afferent nerve fibres linking the peripheral receptor systems in the vertebral and paravertebral tissues with the spinal cord. In this case, the pathological changes are not to be found in the lumbosacral tissues in which the pain is perceived, but somewhere along the course of the afferent nerve fibres that innervate those tissues. Should compressive lesions occur, of which the most obvious example is a posterolateral herniation of the nucleus pulposus of a lumbar intervertebral disc, and if it proves to be progressive, a specific sequence of events in the nerve fibres contained in the lumbosacral nerve roots takes place, which is reflected in the changing phenomena that are presented clinically, as the lesion develops.

Because of the correlation between the diameter of nerve fibres and their metabolic activity, conduction in the larger, mechanoceptor fibres in the spinal nerves is interfered with earlier and more severely by any disturbance of the blood supply than is that in the smaller nociceptor afferent fibres in the same nerves. There is a consequent selective loss of the inhibitory effect of the former on the central, centripetal transsynaptic propagation of activity in the latter system. If such a protrusion develops further, it may not only interrupt mechanoceptor afferent activity, but it may also irritate nociceptive afferent fibres contained in the sinu-vertebral nerve, giving rise to pain in the lower back, in the absence of sciatica. If the protrusion increases more in size, it begins to impinge upon the related dorsal roots and their containing dural sleeves, as a result of which the backache becomes more severe and more widely distributed, being supplemented by concomitant, painful reflex muscle spasm. To this are added the sensory changes of paraesthesiae and numbness.

Thus the initial change is increase in pain sensitivity (especially in response to static and dynamic mechanical forces) of the articular, ligamentous and muscular tissues of the back, as mechanoceptor activity normally derived therefrom is progressively interfered with. As nerve root compression increases, this is followed by intermittent or continuous irritation of the smaller diameter nociceptive afferent fibres in the same nerve roots and their dural sleeves, so that the backache becomes more severe and is less readily relieved by changes in posture or by activity. Compression of the intraspinal nerve roots may persist to the extent that the resulting chronic ischaemia produces degeneration of the mechanoceptive but not the nociceptive afferent fibres carried therein. The backache becomes almost continuous, and its relief by mechanical means becomes increasingly ineffectual.

Referred backache

Pain may be experienced in the lower back, although the causative lesion lies neither in the tissues in which the pain is felt nor along the course of the afferent fibres that innervate these tissues, but instead involves some tissue or organ whose innervation is segmentally related to that of the superficial tissues of the lumbosacral spine; this constitutes referred backache. The development of a primary visceral or peritoneal disorder may be accompanied by pain (and often hyperaesthesia) in one or more sectors of the skin in the lumbosacral area, in which reflex vasomotor changes may also occur, and this is frequently associated with reflex spasm of segmentally related portions of the spinal musculature.

Recent research has thrown considerable light on this phenomenon, especially with the demonstration that nociceptive afferents from visceral tissues project onto the same relay cells in lamina 5 of the basal spinal nucleus as do the afferents from segmentally related areas of the skin. Normal or trivial stimuli applied to these areas may induce these relay cells to fire, should their excitability be sufficiently increased by pre-existing afferent activity emanating from visceral nociceptive nerve endings. The resulting pain is then perceived to lie in the skin.

Clinically, referred backache is most commonly encountered gynaecologically: in dysmenorrhoea, in lesions of the ovaries or of the Fallopian tubes, such as in salpingitis or ectopic pregnancy, or with uterine prolapse or retroversion and, finally, in carcinoma of the uterine cervix. Apart from these, patients with diseases of the urinary tract often experience referred backache, particularly with pyelitis, pyelonephritis and renal calculi. It may also occur in lesions of the renal pelvis, in the presence of a retrocaecal appendix and in various forms of prostatitis.

EXAMINATION

As has already been emphasized, thorough and meticulous examination is essential.

Posture and global movements

One notes kyphosis, scoliosis etc. Pelvic tilt will be discussed below, in the section on the Pelvis. The global movements (flexion, extension, lateroflexion and rotation) are tested. These movements, let it be emphasized, are of relatively little diagnostic value. They are extremely useful in recording clinical progress and therapeutic response.

Neurological examination

This is aimed at eliciting neurological deficit and/or root irritability:

(1) *Muscle power*

plantar-flexion S1
dorsiflexion L5
eversion L5/S1
diffuse weakness – query emotional state

(2) *Referred muscle tenderness*

tender calf S1
tender tibial compartment L5
tender quadriceps L4

(3) *Sensation*

numbness and/or paraesthesiae affecting the medial aspect of:
thigh and calf L4
dorsum of foot L5
lateral aspect of foot S1

(4) *Reflexes*

knee L3/L4
ankle S1

N.B. an absent ankle reflex may be due to a previous episode

(5) *Straight leg raising*

any painful lesion of the back can give a positive straight leg raise

With regard to the neurological examination, the findings of Mooney must be borne in mind[150]. He and his co-workers at present will only accept as true localizing neurological signs sensory changes, specific motor weakness and probably a positive crossed leg straight leg raising test. Moreover, there are considerable reservations to be expressed with regard to the straight leg raising test. Firstly, many structures are involved and further, spasm of hamstrings or hip joint pathology will restrict movement. It is normal for people to vary between 70° and 120°, there is commonly a 10% variation of normal between right and left legs in the same individual and, further, many people develop pain spontaneously at no more than 60°. Finally, not only can straight leg raising be restored to normal by treatment of zygoapophyseal joints, but King, in 1977, by treating trigger spots in the paravertebral musculature, also restored normality[155]. Its principal value seems to be not so much as a diagnostic procedure but as a means of monitoring therapeutic progress.

Palpatory tests

These are described and illustrated in the section on Diagnostic Techniques.

(1)   skin-drag

(2)   skin-rolling

(3)   palpation of the paravertebral muscles

(4)   widespread palpation for tenderness, particularly along the pelvic brim

It should be noted that positive skin-roll over the buttocks frequently indicates thoracolumbar problems. In testing for paravertebral spasm or tenderness, particular attention should be directed to the iliac crests and the area between the spinous process of L5 and the sacrum.

CONVENTIONAL RADIOLOGY

For many years efforts have been made to correlate radiologically demonstrated changes, particularly degenerative, and symptoms. 'Autopsy studies report a considerably higher percentage of the incidence of spondylosis than do clinical radiological studies'[116]. In fact, the relationship between disc degeneration and low back pain is controversial. It is clear 'that disc degeneration *per se* is not symptomatic and is part of a general age process'[16]. Back pain is far more more frequent in subjects over the age of 50 if they have severe disc degeneration at several levels[220]. 'Most other aberrations from the normal in the lumbar area, except spondylolisthesis and severe kyphosis, have been demonstrated with the same incidence in low back patients as in controls. This includes facet tropism and arthrosis'[140]. Indeed, Magora and Schwarz, in 1976, observed that the finding of a single narrow disc occurred more often in the group of people who had never experienced back pain than in those with low back pain[221]. In people with moderate or slight degeneration, most authorities report a negative correlation[220,221]. Further, as we have mentioned elsewhere, the incidence of back pain starts in the twenties, reaches a maximum between the ages of 40 and 50 and diminishes thereafter[140] – this at a time when degenerative changes are continuing, as revealed, *pari passu*, by conventional radiology.

Attempts have also been made to relate back pain to skeletal defects, be they congenital or acquired. La Rocca and Macnab, in 1969, showed that many different defects exist without causing pain[217]. With regard to spondylolisthesis, some authorities have found it to be associated positively with low back pain[222]. However, this is rebutted by others (notably La Rocca and Macnab), and it is impossible to assess the number of persons with spondylolisthesis in the general population, since so many of them are asymptomatic[217]. Sorenson also showed that despite the opinions of many persons, there is no positive correlation between back pain and Scheuermann's disease and severe lumbar scoliosis[223]. Nor is there with sacralization or spina bifida[224]. Finally, while it is known that vertebral and osteoporosis can be painful in middle-aged or young subjects, positive correlation has not been shown [217,220].

Every general practitioner will be familiar with the patient who has been told by another clinician that because of degenerative changes in his spine, shown radiologically, his back pain is fixed and there is little or nothing anyone can do for him. In view of the above material, this is simply not so. One of the real contributions lay manipulators make at the present time arises from the fact that the medical profession is insufficiently alerted as to how common vertebral problems are and how to diagnose and treat them. While this may or may not be regrettable, it is certainly sad that the lay manipulator may be the only hope for a patient who has been given the advice outlined above. The solution to the problems which still dominate the field of musculoskeletal medicine will ultimately come from the stables of orthodox academic neurology, orthopaedics and rheumatology. Indeed, it is interesting to observe how much clinically relevant material has come from these sources over the last few years. It is disturbing, however, that this material has often not reached people engaged in clinical practice, especially general practice. The use made of the degenerative X-ray of the lumbar spine is perhaps the most striking example of this phenomenon.

LUMBAR INJECTIONS

1. Trigger-point injections

These points are sought in the tissues around vertebral joints. They may also be found in the leg muscles. The commonest site is in the midline between L4 and S1.

Indications
The finding of such points requires particularly thorough palpation. Although the explanation is ill-understood, the injection of such a point in a patient with back and leg pain may relieve all his symptoms. Thus Steindler and Luck, in 1938, assessed 451 cases of low back pain with referred pain to the leg on localized palpation in the lumbosacral region[54]. Of these cases, 228 were relieved, by lumbosacral injection of local anaesthetic, both of local and of referred pain.

2. Nerve blocks

These are rarely used in general practice. In view of the phenomenon of pain of spinal origin simulating visceral disease, however, the work of Ashby in 1977 is of great interest[206]. In 73 patients presenting with abdominal pain in the course of a year, he was able to relieve the symptoms by spinal nerve blocks. Meralgia paraesthetica is an entrapment neuropathy of the lateral femoral cutaneous nerve as it emerges from under the inguinal ligament, causing anaesthesia, paraesthesiae or pain on the anterolateral aspect of the thigh. Some doubt has been thrown upon the existence of traditional diagnosis by the work of Dan in 1976[225]. Observing that many of these patients had marked lordosis, he prescribed flexion exercises and advice to improve the patients' posture with considerable success. It may well be, therefore, that the cause of symptoms is more central than peripheral. The technique used is to infiltrate 5 cc of local steroids widely at the site of emergence, as the site of emergence is variable.

3. Attachment tissue injections

These are of the greatest importance in low back pain. The structures most commonly injected are the supra- and interspinous ligaments, the tissue attachments to the pelvic brim and the tips of the transverse processes. Ingpen and Burry, in 1970, claimed marked success by using one or two injections combined with lumbar isometric exercises[149]. The site of injection was the area of maximum tenderness between the 5th lumbar spinous process and the posterior superior iliac spine. They used a combination of local anaesthetic and steroids.

Technique
Using a solution of 5 ml of 1% lignocaine and 5 ml of hydrocortisone, half is deposited at the site of maximum tenderness and the residue around it. The solution employed may be varied by the individual physician.

4. Apophyseal joints

These are now widely recognized as being a potential source of low back pain and sciatica and their injection with local steroids and anaesthetic is becoming increasingly common. In 1974, Shealey used this injection as a diagnostic procedure with a view to going on to subsequent apophyseal joint rhizolysis[226]. In the same year Burnell noted that injections could diminish symptoms in apophyseal joints and the immediate prescription of active exercises could frequently have beneficial results[154]. It was then observed that many of these patients had their symptoms relieved and, therefore, rhizolysis was no longer necessary. In 1976, Mooney found that on injecting hypertonic saline into the apophyseal joints, the straight leg raising was limited to 70°, there was marked myeloelectrical activity in the hamstring muscles and, in 15% of cases, depression of tendon reflexes[52]. All these findings were subsequently reversed by steroid injections. The implications for traditional neurological examination need no emphasis. In 1977, Mooney and Robertson subsequently went on to investigate

100 patients[150]. 'Each complained of lumbago or sciatica clinically indistinguishable from "the disc syndrome". Referred pain from apophyseal joints was induced in the low back, buttock, groin and leg and obliterated by injection of 2–5 ml of 1% xylocaine. ... Initial experience with the use of radiologically confirmed injection of steroids and local anaesthetic into the facet joint has suggested that this regime alone may give long-term relief in 20% of back pain sufferers and partial relief in 30%'[227].

The technique is to have the patient lying prone, when a tender area is sought by deep palpation one finger's breadth lateral to the spinous process. This is an accurate locating method, as radio-opaque markers placed on these spots have been shown radiologically to overlie the apophyseal joints[91]. 5 ml of local anaesthetic plus 5 ml of steroids are used with a 2-inch (5 cm) needle. Occasionally, in obese or muscular patients, a longer needle is necessary. 5 ml are deposited in the vicinity of the joint – 2·5 ml deposited $1\frac{1}{2}$ inches (4 cm) above, and the residue $1\frac{1}{2}$ inches (4 cm) below.

5.   Epidural analgesia via the sacral hiatus (caudal epidural)

Caussade and Chauffard used this technique in the treatment of sciatica as long ago as 1909[228].

Indication

The technique is indicated in very severe lumbago, agonizing sciatica, chronic sciatica or differential diagnosis[229].

   Epidural analgesia will be produced in:

(1)   structures innervated by the sinu-vertebral nerve,
(2)   the nerve sheath,
(3)   the dura mater,
(4)   the posterior longitudinal ligament,
(5)   the apophyseal joint.

Therefore, it will be seen that this technique may be of value in situations where the diagnosis is by no means certain.

Solutions employed

Cyriax concluded that the addition of steroid to local anaesthetic was of no assistance[230].

Yates, comparing four differing solutions, proved that the addition of steroid had a significant advantage in the restoration of mobility[228].

This discrepancy of view reinforces our statement as to the difficulty in establishing any clear preference regarding the materials to be used in these and other vertebral injections.

Technique

With the patient prone, a $1\frac{1}{2}$-inch (4 cm) needle is introduced into the epidural space, and the solution injected at the rate of 5–10 ml per minute (illustrated in Chapter 9).

Volume

This is very variable. We use 20 ml. 40 ml or over is potentially dangerous.

Value

Harley, in 50 successive cases of sciatica using one or two injections, achieved complete relief in 20 cases, improvement in 13 and no change in 17[231].

In 1961, Coomes investigated two groups of 20 patients with severe sciatica[232]. One group was treated by caudal epidurals and the other by bed rest. Symptoms before treatment were similar in duration, 37 days for the group having epidurals and 31 days for those having bed rest. Solutions used were 50 ml of $\frac{1}{2}\%$ procaine. The average recovery time for the group having bed rest was 31 days and for injection 11 days. The injected group also had a greater improvement in 'neurological' signs than did the other.

Dangers

These are minimal, potential problems are local sepsis, sensitivity to the anaesthetic and excessive volume.

Comment

In an area where precise diagnosis is often difficult and sometimes impossible, this is an extremely valuable diagnostic therapeutic tool.

It is worth noting that, according to Professor Wyke, less than 5% of patients presenting with low back pain have prolapse of the nucleus pulposus[215]. In view of the importance of this statement, it is worth giving the references here[233–238].

THE PELVIS

Very little is known about the pelvis – far less than is known about the spine, because surgical information concerning the latter is available whereas intervention with regard to the bony pelvis is extremely rare. Physiologically, however, the pelvis is perfectly capable of mediating pain and there is no reason to suppose it is unique in not doing so. The symptoms of pain present the same difficulties we have encountered with regard to the spine, examination presents problems of its own.

Applied anatomy of the sacro-iliac joints

Joint surfaces are grossly irregular and so formed that there are at least two and often three surfaces angulated to one another. Differences between the joints in the same individual are common. Solonen found variations in 25 out of 30 specimens[239]. In only five were the two sacro-iliac joints alike.

Movement

It has been assumed in the past that sacro-iliac joint movement consists primarily of rotation occurring around a fixed mechanical axis. In 1955, Weisl showed by cineradiography that in rotation the axis lies about 10 cm below the sacral promontory and is *variable* by about 5 cm[240]. Colachis, in 1963, inserted Kirschner pins into the iliac spines of medical students[241]. The movements of individuals vary greatly, there is no fixed axis and angular and parallel movements take place rather more than rotation. In 1974, it was shown that any sacral movement is associated with correlated antagonistic movements of both ilia[242]. On flexing both hip and knee it can be shown that in the unsupported limb the posterior superior iliac spine rotates backwards and that the ischial tuberosity moves laterally.

Asymmetry of the pelvis

Bony asymmetry of the ilia is common. Lewit observed 450 school-children and found that 40% had asymmetry[243]. There was no positive clinical correlation between asymmetry and symptoms. Leg length again presents the same problems. Asymmetry frequently exists without symptoms; symptoms frequently exist without asymmetry. Symptoms combined with asymmetry can be treated by manipulation. Commonly the symptoms disappear, but in the majority of cases the asymmetry remains. In view of the above, the classic system of osteopathic diagnosis assuming pure rotation during movements and alterations in juxtaposition of the bony points of the pelvis to be detectable seems untenable. Its survival is probably due to the effectiveness of treatment. People are more likely to question the means by which they arrive at a diagnosis in the presence of clinical failure rather than success.

The joint is too deep and the movement too slight to make detection of hypermobility or hypomobility other than subjective. With the patient supine bringing the flexed knee into adduction then towards the contralateral shoulder and then the ipsilateral shoulder is said to stress in sequence the ilio-lumbar, sacro-iliac and sacrotuberous ligaments. Many other structures are stretched in the course of this movement. In short, signs implicating individual sacro-iliac joints are unreliable. How is one to conduct an examination, therefore, in practice?

(1) Conduct a *full* examination of the lumbar spine and hip. Problems of the lumbar spine and hip can, of course, coexist with pelvic lesions.

(2) Iliac 'gapping' and approximation.

(3) Pressure over the sacral apex.

(4) Pressure over the symphysis pubis.

(5) Palpation particularly over the posterior inferior iliac spine. The whole area should be palpated, bearing in mind the phenomenon of referred tenderness. Finding a positive sign should lead to manipulation, in the absence of contraindications. Some therapeutic techniques are more effective than others, but it

must be remembered that any manipulation of the pelvic joints affects the lower lumbar spine also. Success, therefore, does not exclude the spine from being the cause of the problem.

(6) Differences in movement of the sacro-iliac joints may be discernible, using a simple test. With the patient prone, the tips of the third and fourth fingers of one hand press firmly down over the sacrum just medial to the posterior superior iliac spine, abutting on its medial aspect. The fingers of the other hand are used to 'rock' the anterior superior iliac spine gently. Movement against the palpating fingers is felt in the majority of cases and the two sides compared. This test has value only in monitoring change in mobility following treatment.

Conclusion

While the pelvis certainly is the source of pain at times, diagnosis is far from satisfactory at present. Nevertheless, success of manipulation is such that, given safety by careful observation of the contra-indications and the use of suitable techniques, it is clearly to the patient's advantage.

THE INTERVERTEBRAL DISC

Despite the fact that Wyke, in 1976, considered it should be emphasized that less than 5% of patients with backache had prolapsed intervertebral discs, this subject merits a presentation on its own in view of the enormous volume of literature associated with it over the last 50 years[215].

In 1932, a Dr Barr of Massachusetts was the first person to appreciate that material recently removed from one of his patients as a chondroma was in reality a herniated disc[244]. 'He solved one important part of the low back pain problem but, as we all know by now, it was only a minor part'[141]. After Barr's discovery, the diagnosis of prolapsed intervertebral disc was made on an enormous scale. Disc problems were considered by many to be almost the universal cause of low back pain. The most prominent proponent of this school in the present day is probably Dr Cyriax. It is a diagnosis still very commonly made in general practice. An indication of the hold it has seized over the clinical mind is that over 3000 papers have been published on this subject in the period since World War II alone. Arnoldi, in 1972, wrote, 'pain in the lumbar area can originate in a number of differently structured elements and if we accept the apparently clear cut syndromes with nerve root affection caused by disc herniation, we cannot say that our understanding has gained substantially from the impressive pool of detailed information'[245].

'It is apparent that causes of compression of the cauda equina and nerve roots other than single disc protrusions, are much more common than previously thought. Some authors are of the opinion that these other causes are responsible for two thirds of the patients' [246]).

In a series of 227 patients who came to surgery, only 70 had a single prolapse of the nucleus pulposus, 65 had lumbar spondylosis and five stenosis. The remainder had combinations of two or more of these factors.

Thus there is no clinical sign or combinations of signs which prove diagnosis of a disc protrusion other than those of a space-occupying lesion.

The history

Duration and progression of symptoms
The sudden onset of pain following provocative activity and subsequently an intermittent course related to activity is highly suggestive of a mechanical problem[43].

Site and radiation
The history of site and radiation of pain is of little help in indicating the structure or structures in which the pain originates. Pain due to root irritation may spread to the thigh, calf and even the foot. Such pain is frequently associated with paraesthesiae or numbness involving the lateral border of the foot in an S1 lesion and the dorsum of the foot and the leg if L5 is involved.

Activities
Close questioning concerning the disability and the activities of daily living are important for two reasons: firstly, a correlation between symptoms and activities provides an assessment of the emotional

status of the patient, and secondly it provides a means of monitoring therapeutic response.

Examination
(1) Posture
    (a) query kyphosis?
    (b) query scoliosis?

(2) Global movements
    (a) flexion
    (b) extension
    (c) lateroflexion
    (d) rotation

(3) Neurology
    (a) *Reflexes*
      knee   L3/L4
      ankle   S1
    (b) *Power*
      dorsiflexors of the foot   L5
      flexor hallucis longus   S1
    (c) *Sensation*
      anteromedial aspect of the thigh   L4
      dorsum of the foot   L5
      outer border of leg and foot   S1
    (d) *Referred tenderness*
      tender quadriceps   L4
      tender tibial muscles   L5
      tender calf   S1

(4) Straight leg raising. *See* section on lumbar examination, above

(5) The hip. Full examination is essential, as the hip can produce symptoms in identical distribution

(6) *Special investigations.* With regard to special investigations, myelography, radiculography, CAT scanning and ultrasound have been used. With regard to myelography, however, Hitselberger, in 1969, using this procedure to investigate 300 asymptomatic individuals found a positive myelogram in 37% of cases and strongly positive in 9%[114]. Hudgins, bearing in mind that

up to 20% of myelograms are negative in the presence of a positive disc, regarded a positive crossed leg extensor test as an indication for surgery even in the absence of a positive myelogram[247]. Lansche in an exhaustive study on the surgical confirmation of positive myelograms, found accuracy in only 39.2%[248]. Therefore, the use of special investigations presents difficulties. This is emphasized in the preoperative selection of cases of which a typical system is that of Finneson and Cooper, who used a points score[249]. Thus disc problems outline the principal difficulty we all have in low back problems, which is that of accurate diagnosis.

Clinical importance of the dura mater

With regard to the dura mater, it is necessary to clear up a longstanding neurological fallacy. For many years, it has been assumed by many authorities that compression or irritation of afferent fibres entering the spinal cord in the dorsal roots causes pain referred peripherally down the leg. This is not so, as the compression of a peripheral nerve *never* produces pain in the distribution of that nerve. So-called sciatica can be due to two factors. Firstly, in the presence of a degenerated disc, enzymatic digestion of proteoglycans takes place. The breakdown products of these proteoglycans are intensely irritant to nociceptors and can therefore irritate the dural sleeve, which is why referred pain in sciatica is dural in distribution. Secondly, compression of the dural sleeve will produce pain, again in the distribution of dural referred pain. A further factor operates, however. The larger fibres are more physiologically active and require a greater blood supply. If this supply is impaired by compression, the larger fibres will be affected before the smaller ones. These fibres contain afferents from mechanoceptors Types 1, 2 and 3, therefore this will distort the picture further and more pain will ensue[4].

Treatment

Manipulation may be helpful if symptoms and signs are relatively slight. If either or both are severe, a favourable response is unlikely and the manoeuvre may well be painful. If it proves painful, it should be abandoned, but pain-free manipulation commonly produces surprisingly good results and should not be eschewed.

5
Peripheral Joints

THE SHOULDER

Introduction

This presentation is deliberately simplified with a view to affording the generalist a straightforward and effective system for dealing with shoulder problems. Thus, such matters as posture are omitted less by ignorance than by design. It must be remembered that examination of the cervical spine and of the contralateral shoulder are essential preliminaries.

Relevant anatomy

(1) The extreme mobility, due to a combination of factors, including the shallowness of the glenoid cavity (by contrast, say with the hip)

(2) The unique maintenance of stability by its surrounding tendons. The biceps holding the humeral head into the glenoid cavity. The reinforcement of the joint capsule by subscapularis and supraspinous and teres minor posteriorly. The 'rotator cuff'

(3) Upward movement of the humeral head is limited by a fibro-osseous arch between acromion and corocoid processes, which form the roof of the shoulder joint

(4) Between this arch and the rotator cuff lies the subacromial bursa which *often* communicates with the main joint cavity

Medical orthopaedics

The peculiar anatomy of the joint perhaps explains the particular stresses the tissues about it sustain, and hence the frequency of

problems that result. There is a group of conditions (supraspinatus tendinitis and/or calcification, rotator cuff lesions, subacromial bursitis,
capsulitis, frozen shoulder) which are common, but anatomically and
pathologically not clearly understood. They are all closely interrelated. Thus, subacromial bursitis is generally considered to follow on
problems affecting the supraspinatus tendon. This, being relatively
avascular and poorly innervated, can be inflamed but pain-free until
the neighbouring bursa, being abundantly supplied with nerves and
blood vessels, is affected[250]. Again, with a frozen shoulder, not only
the capsule, but all periarticular structures show abnormalities. These
problems can and should be diagnosed and treated in general practice[251].

While the cause is unknown, it must be remembered that the
frozen shoulder can have not only local causes but occurs:

(1) in connection with ischaemic heart disease or chronic pulmon-
     ary disease,

(2) following a neurological lesion, particularly hemiplegia or
     herpes zoster,

(3) following intrathoracic surgery or operations of the breast.

Examination

Inspection
Occasionally, there is some evidence of swelling with subacromial
bursitis.

Neck
The detailed examination of the neck, and its treatment if indicated,
is essential. One third of arm pain is cervical in origin. It is relevant
even if shoulders have painful and restricted movements.

Capsule
Active and passive movements are:

   hand to neck
   hand to back
   abduction
   anterior elevation

Analysis of results

(1) Restriction of active movements merely indicates a shoulder and possibly a neck problem.

(2) Restriction of passive movements is of capital importance.

  (a) The capsular pattern: generally restricted and painful movements (capsulitis) or extremely restricted but less painful movements (frozen shoulder).

  (b) The non-capsular pattern: marked limitation and pain on abduction (subacromial bursitis)[252].

(3) The painful arc: pain elicited on abduction between 60° and 120° is assumed to be due to an inflamed supraspinatus tendon pressing on the acromion above. Lack of pain on external rotation and then abduction of the arm reinforces this impression.

(4) Passive abduction: the scapula must be fixed during this movement to elicit true glenohumeral, and not total shoulder, movement.

Cuff

Resisted movements are[252]:

  abduction – deltoid and supraspinatus
  adduction – pectoralis major and teres minor and major
  external rotation – infraspinatus and teres minor
  internal rotation – subscapularis
  flexion and supination at the elbow – biceps

Analysis

Pain on resisted movements indicates that a cuff lesion may exist, no more. Bicipital tendinitis can exist without pain on resisted supination and flexion.

Palpation is all-important. It will elicit a lesion that resisted movements may not and indicates the site for treatment. It is assessed by comparison with the contralateral shoulder, which must invariably be examined first.

Acromioclavicular and sternoclavicular joints

The symptoms are invariably localized, thus simplifying matters.

Acromioclavicular joint
Movements: active and passive shoulder movements are full and are painful at the extremes, notably on adduction. Palpation reveals local tenderness and sometimes subluxation.

Sternoclavicular joint
Active and passive movements may cause slight discomfort, particularly on adduction. Palpation will reveal tenderness and rarely subluxation.

Treatment

(1) Manipulation has no place in treatment of the shoulder. Performed under general anaesthesia, it is capable of producing severe and prolonged reaction.

(2) Injection.

177

   (a) Injection of steroids into joint capsule is frequently of great benefit in acute capsulitis, its efficacy in chronic capsulitis being much less. Therefore, early diagnosis and treatment is important.

   (b) In subacromial bursitis, injection of steroids under the arch of the acromion, using the lateral approach, is extremely useful.

   (c) In rotator cuff lesions, injections should be directed primarily at such sites of tenderness as are detected.

(3) Drugs may be employed: analgesics and/or anti-inflammatories may be of value, depending upon individual response.

(4) Ultrasound may be valuable in acute lesions, though much less so in established cases.

(5) Acupuncture, although still a matter of contention, may be of substantial help in resistant cases, as may transcutaneous nerve stimulation.

THE ELBOW, WRIST AND HAND

Elbow

Anatomically, the elbow is a joint complex with articulations between humerus, radius and ulna, which are so designed as to permit flexion, extension, supination and pronation, coupled with considerable stability. This is achieved in one synovial 'package' by virtue of the shape and positioning of the articular components, coupled with the curvature of the radial and ulnar shafts. The inferior end of the humerus is angled anteriorly to nearly 45°, while the trochlear notch of the ulna faces both anteriorly and superiorly, permitting the olecranon process to fit into the olecranon fossa in extension. The trochlea of the humerus, pulley-shaped, accepts the trochlear notch of the ulna, which has two corresponding articular surfaces, permitting a true hinge action. The capitulum, hemispherical, accepts the concave radial head, much of which is bevelled so as to engage with the capitulo-trochlear groove, permitting the radius to join in the flexion/extension movements of the ulna and to rotate within the joint formed between the rim of its head and the fibro-osseous ring, the latter composed of the radial notch of the ulna and the annular ligament.

Special features relating to the elbow are three: (1) the olecranon bursa, commonly the site of traumatic effusion, (2) the flexor attachment tissues, giving rise to golfer's elbow, and (3) the extensor attachment tissues giving rise to tennis elbow.

Fractures of the olecranon or of the radial head are relatively uncommon, dislocation of the radial head perhaps rather less common (in tears of the annular ligament), while distal humeral fractures are again uncommon. All are surgical problems, and their importance depends largely on whether or not the fracture involves the synovial joint-complex.

Wear and tear of osteoarthrosis are common and are characterized by loss of articular cartilage and of joint space, with bony sclerosis. Rheumatoid arthritis is fairly common, with loss of cartilage and of joint space, but with areas of localized porosis and with breaches of bony cortex, and, in advanced cases, gross disorganization of the joint. Infective arthritis of the elbow is rare.

In practice, the orthopaedic physician will most commonly need to treat olecranon bursitis and the attachment tissue injuries. Bursitis requires aspiration and firm support (e.g. crepe bandage) and, if infected, adequate antibiotic therapy. Injection of attachment tissues in tennis elbow and golfer's elbow with a mixture of local anaesthetic and steroid is frequently indicated in practice, the results often being so good as to obviate any indication for manipulation. Deep transverse friction may work, but is unkind to the patient, is hard work for the physiotherapist and takes very much longer than injections. Pulled elbow and some cases of attachment tissue injury may well benefit from ultrasound or interferential therapy.

Wrist and hand

The wrist is a joint complex, which may be regarded as a universal soft-tissue coupling, reinforced by bony components. This implies a limited movement in any direction. This view is supported by the synovial system, which is common to all joints of the wrist, and it is really misleading to consider each joint separately.

The distal radio-ulnar joint moves very little, as most of the supination/pronation of the forearm is performed by rotation of the radial head within the annular ligament, the curvature of the radius permitting it to swing round the ulna.

The radiocarpal joint, which includes the carpal disc (which separates the ulna styloid from the wrist joint proper), is between the radius and the scaphoid, lunate and triquetrum. The scaphoid articulates distally with the trapezium and trapezoid. The lunate articulates proximally with the radius and the carpal disc, laterally with the scaphoid, medially with the triquetrum and distally with the capitate only. The triquetrum articulates proximally with the carpal disc, laterally with the lunate, medially with the pisiform (the only joint involving the latter), and distally with the hamate. The distal articulations of the scaphoid, lunate and triquetrum constitute the midcarpal joint.

The carpometacarpal joints are peculiar in that the first metacarpal articulates with the trapezium, the second with both the trapezium and trapezoid, the third with the capitate, the fourth with fibrous tissue only between capitate and hamate, the fifth with the hamate alone.

The features special to the wrist and hand are the carpal tunnel,

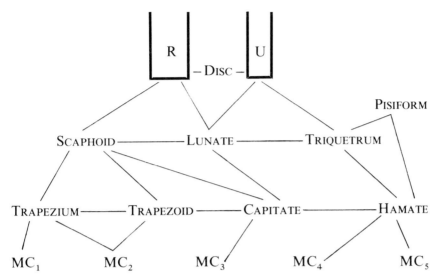

Diagrammatic representation of articulations of the wrist

housing flexor tendons, blood vessels, and the median nerve, the flexor sheaths and the palmar spaces. The problems are traumatic, those due to unaccustomed or excessive activity (e.g. tenosynovitis), inflammatory or infective. The traumatic include Colles and Smith fractures, scaphoid fractures and those of the metacarpals and phalanges; also sprains of the associated joint capsules and supporting ligaments. The next group includes tenosynovitis and the carpal tunnel syndrome. Wear and tear appears as in the elbow, with the appearance of Heberden's nodes, rheumatoid arthritis presenting typically, the most diagnostically difficult being the early cases. Infective arthritides are rare, as are palmar space infections.

Fractures must be referred to the surgeons, unless the doctor has appropriate facilities. Sprains require heat or cold or both, ultrasound, support bandaging, or analgesics, with or without anti-inflammatories. Simple subluxations require reduction prior to other treatment. Rheumatoid arthritis requires referral to the rheumatologists and infections need to be treated primarily with antibiotics, although palmar space infections may require surgical drainage. Tenosynovitis requires immobilization, adequate analgesia, and anaesthetic/steroid injection. Carpal tunnel syndrome, *after exclusion of a cervical spinal origin*, demands anaesthetic/steroid injection, which is commonly effective, with referral of the 'failures' to the orthopaedic surgeons.

THE HIP

Introduction

Pain of vertebral origin is frequently referred to the area of the hip joint. The fact that hip pain can be referred to buttock, groin, thigh, knee, and as far as the ankle, means that the examination of this joint is mandatory in every case of lumbago and sciatica. It is, however, frequently neglected.

Examination

Gait
Gait with or without a walking stick can be informative. The Trendelenburg test is performed by observation of the relative heights of the two anterosuperior iliac spines while the patient stands first on one leg and then on the other. Normally, the pelvis tilts upwards on the non-weight-bearing side. Weight-bearing on a diseased hip may produce the opposite effect.

Palpation
The depth of the joint from the surface means that joint effusions, swelling and local tenderness are much less apparent than with more superficial joints. Nevertheless, deep palpation over the middle of the inguinal ligament (i.e. over the front of the joint) and above the greater trochanter (i.e. over the piriformis) can be informative. In suspected hip disease, abdominal examination is frequently indicated.

Leg length
Some estimation of leg length may be of value. This has been reviewed in Chapter 4, in the section on the Pelvis.

Flexion (115°)
With the patient supine, the flexed knee is brought towards the abdomen. The knee must be flexed to avoid a 'sciatic stretch' effect,

and the angle recorded is that at which further flexion produces pelvic tilting. It is important to remember that a flexion deformity of the hip can be masked by pelvic tilting. Such a compensatory lumbar lordosis can be abolished by fully flexing the opposite hip joint (confirmed by a hand over the upper sacrum), and this will make apparent any fixed flexion deformity.

Extension (30°)
With the patient lying on the opposite side, the observer, from behind, draws the leg backwards. The angle recorded is that at which any further movement is achieved by pelvic tilting. An assistant is essential for this test if the subject is disabled.

Abduction (50°)
With the patient supine, the leg is carried outwards. For serial measurements, the 'total straddle' can be recorded as the distance between the medial malleoli when both hips are abducted.

Abduction (45°)
The technique is similar to abduction, except that the leg is carried medially in front of the opposite limb.

Rotation (internal 45°, external 45°)
This may be tested with the leg in the standard zero starting position (which amounts to rolling the leg from the side on the couch), or with the hip flexed to 90°. In practice, there is not much difference in the results obtained, and many clinicians find the 90° position most convenient. However, with the leg straight, the test is more sensitive.

Individual variation
It must be appreciated that the figures given are approximate and that normal movement of all joints varies considerably between individuals.

Hip problems

Paediatric
All these conditions are serious, and diagnosis depends substantially on radiology. Any child with positive symptoms and signs should be put to bed straight away until the cause is established.

Perthes' disease

This is a unilateral or bilateral osteochondrosis affecting boys between the ages of 4 and 12 years. Trivial pain is felt in thigh or knee,
the child limps, and examination reveals marked limitation of movements of the hip joint. X-rays show flattening of the femoral head so
that it does not fit the acetabulum. Long-term osteoarthrosis is probable.

Slipped femoral epiphysis

For reasons not understood, at around the age of 12, usually in the
female, the epiphyseal junction and the femoral head can slip on the
neck of the femur. Early diagnosis is important and immediate orthopaedic referral indicated.

Congenital dislocation

This has an incidence of 12 in 10 000 in girls, and two in 10 000 for
boys. Routine post-natal examination should include Ortalani's test
(flexion, abduction and seeking excessive joint-play), as early diagnosis and treatment avoids long-term osteoarthrosis.

Adult problems

Osteoarthrosis

This is an exceedingly important condition. Its diagnosis is clinical,
and the radiological appearances have no positive correlation with
the severity of the symptoms. Treatment is difficult. Initial analgesic
or anti-inflammatory agents may have to give way to steroid injections. Frequently, the piriformis is tender over the greater trochanter,
and injection of this muscle often gives prolonged relief, without the
anxieties of injecting steroid into the synovial cavity of a weight-
bearing joint. Failure leads ultimately to surgery.

Place of exercises in osteoarthrosis

Non-weight-bearing exercises may be of substantial value, particularly in early cases. In the continuing presence of the arthrosis,
these must be continued for life.

THE KNEE AND ANKLE

Knee

Cartilage problems

The medial cartilage is involved several times more frequently than the lateral. The typical history is of a rotation sprain of a weight-bearing flexed knee, as in football. Of great importance from the point of view of treatment is: if an effusion develops, how quickly after the incident does this happen. If this occurs in minutes rather than hours, the likelihood of blood in the joint is very great.

Treatment is as follows.

(1) Manipulation if it is 'locked', as soon after injury as possible. This is performed with the knee flexed, abducted, externally rotated and then extended. If manipulation cannot be done without anaesthesia, early orthopaedic referral is obviously necessary.

(2) Effusion. If this is haemorrhagic, it must be dealt with by aspiration as soon as possible. Following this, a crepe bandage is applied daily until the knee is pain-free.

Medial and lateral ligament sprain

The former is frequent; the latter is rare.

The ideal initial treatment is ultrasound. If pain and tenderness persist after swelling has subsided, local steroids are indicated.

Bursitis

There are several bursae about the knee, the most commonly involved being the prepatellar.

Initially, treatment is aspiration and, in the absence of infection, local steroids. If the condition presents later, i.e. with a solid or semisolid haematoma, ultrasound will be necessary, although of limited value.

Chondromalacia patellae

This can be diagnosed by obtaining crepitus in the usual way and pain on the patient standing from the squatting position. This is a condition found quite frequently in young adults. It is episodic with a good prognosis.

The episodes can normally be controlled with anti-inflammatory medication and surgical referral is rare.

Osteoarthrosis

This often presents in practice as an acute episode.

In this event steroids can be extremely useful injected into the joint capsule and neighbouring tissues at the site of maximum tenderness. It may prove necessary to inject steroids into the joint cavity, in which case frequency of this procedure must be carefully considered, as this is a weight-bearing joint. The maximum number of injections into the joint is three.

Pellegrini–Stieda disease

This is defined as a post-traumatic para-articular osteoma. It presents as a tender, painful swelling of the medial condyle, with characteristic X-ray changes.

Treatment is as follows.

(1) Prophylactic. If the original injury is adequately treated, the formation of an osteoma can be avoided.

(2) If established, masterly inactivity is recommended, since resolution of symptoms will take place in 2–6 months.

Chondrocalcinosis

This is crystal deposition disease in which pyrophosphate crystals are present in the synovial fluid with radiological stippling of the cartilages.

Steroid injection into the joint can be dramatically effective.

Acquired flat feet

Due to descent of the tibia relative to the fibula, there may be minor subluxation of the proximal tibiofibular joint, with laxity of its supporting ligaments.

Treatment is to move the fibular head postero-inferiorly.

Ankle

The commonest lesion of the ankle is a sprain. Ultrasound should be used as soon as possible, for reasons both scientific and psychological. A common problem is the recurring minor sprain following initial resolution. The structures involved can be several but the precise anatomy is not important, since in practice one merely infiltrates with steroids the area or areas of tenderness on palpation. Strapping with Elastoplast may be helpful, provided it relieves tension on the damaged ligaments.

Traumatic arthrosis (McMurray's (1936) 'Footballer's ankle')

Repeated trauma may cause pain, tenderness, and, if the condition evolves, exostosis. Treatment consists primarily of rest. If this fails, surgery can be considered.

Tendo achilles problems

Complete rupture is an important diagnosis. Typically it follows trauma in middle age with local pain, tenderness and swelling. This may be so great as to obscure the rupture. The key test is, with the patient lying prone, to compress the calf muscles causing passive plantar flexion[253]. If negative, urgent orthopaedic referral is indicated.

Partial rupture is a rarity and is usually called a rupture of the plantaris tendon, a diagnosis regarded with universal reservation. Treatment is conservative, unless ultrasound is available. Steroid injection is contraindicated.

Post-traumatic bursitis

This may occur superficial or deep to the tendo achillis, or a subcutaneous adventitious bursa may develop over the calcaneus. This condition, 'winter heel', is associated with ill-fitting footwear. Diagnosis is made by palpation. Treatment is conservative, mainly rest. Local steroids can be useful, but care and accuracy is required as the tendon must not be injected. Occasionally surgery is necessary.

THE FOOT

The foot carries the greatest loads standing and moving. It is the furthest from the heart, and therefore is the coldest part of the body. It is served by the most peripheral of peripheral nerves. Clinically, it has tended to receive relatively scant attention by comparison with, say, the hand.

Hallux valgus

This can be defined as 'a complex progressive deformity affecting the forefoot in which lateral deviation of the great toe is the most obvious feature'[254].

Presenting throughout life, 90% of cases coming to surgery are female. Clinical features are pain felt medially or laterally to the metatarsophalangeal joint or, sometimes, dorsally. Shoe problems are a feature, the patient often being unable to find one wide enough and, as a corollary, cosmetic problems frequently are a presenting complaint. The characteristic deformity is obvious, but other signs (hammer toe, metatarsalgia) must also be sought. The use of splints, insoles and physiotherapy have been well tried in the past, with a uniform lack of success[255]. Surgical shoes with a broad deep toe can be useful. Failure, alas all too common, leads to surgical referral.

Hallux rigidus

This is a painful limitation of dorsiflexion of the metatarsophalangeal joint of the big toe. This presents as either a predominantly female adolescent group, or as an adult group where the sexes are equally divided. The patient typically presents with intermittent acute bouts of pain at the base of the big toe aggravated by walking, particularly in high-heeled shoes. On examination, dorsiflexion is limited and in acute cases all movements are painful. Modification of the shoe with a rocker sole helps in acute cases, although it is difficult to persuade the female adolescent of its use. Injection, in acute cases, of local anaesthetic plus steroid into the joint can be helpful, as can a below-knee walking cast. Failure leads to surgery.

The sole of the foot

Callosities are painful areas of hyperkeratosis usually seen related to one of the downward bony prominences of the foot, i.e. the condition may be due to a mechanical fault. The commonest site is under the metatarsal heads, and therefore symptoms may be relieved by metatarsal domes. Surgery may be necessary.

The plantar fascia

1. Plantar fasciitis

This is a common cause of heel pain in adults of both sexes which is aggravated by weight-bearing and may be severe. On inspection, there is nothing abnormal to be seen, but on palpation there is a point of acute discomfort, usually just forward of the larger medial plantar tubercle of the calcaneus. The nature of the lesion is obscure, but it is assumed to be akin to 'tennis elbow'. Radiological changes are not clinically relevant. Treatment is by sponge rubber heels if local steroid injection fails.

2. Dupuytren's contracture

This can, interestingly enough, be plantar as well as palmar with an incidence of 50%. Clinically, because disabling contractures do not occur, the matter does not present serious problems and is of academic interest.

3. Anterior foot strain

This presents with a vague discomfort of the forefoot on walking a short distance. The physical signs are equally vague, but full passive movements are resented. Its cure is the disruption of fibrous adhesions across the inter metatarsal–phalangeal bursae. The treatment is vigorous restoration of passive movements by manipulation, followed by exercises.

4. Stress fractures

Stress fractures affecting the 2nd, 3rd and 4th metatarsal shafts are common causes of pain. There is usually a gradual onset of pain and swelling of the foot which is aggravated by activity and relieved by rest. One can often palpate a definite swelling in the line of the shaft. An initial X-ray may appear normal, but one taken 2–3 weeks later, however, will show callus. Treatment is to reduce the general level of physical activity and to support-splint the forefoot if necessary.

5. Morton's metatarsalgia

This is a painful lesion, occurring mainly in young or middle-aged women, of the plantar digital nerve where it divides to supply the adjacent sides of a cleft, usually 3/4. Severe pain is felt under the middle of the forefoot usually with radiation into one or more of the three central toes. The pain is absent on waking, but comes on after walking, particularly in tight-fitting footwear. The only helpful sign is pain on pressure upwards and backwards in the web over the point of division of the nerve. Minor cases can be controlled by open types of footwear and limitation of weight-bearing activity, otherwise surgery is indicated.

6. Toes

The 'hammer toe' is a flexion deformity which cannot be overcome by simple stretching. Conservative measures have no place in its treatment.

7. The foot in systemic disorders

Age is the commonest systemic disorder. Clark found that 50% to 80% of adults had something wrong with their feet[256]. Full history and examination with all ancillary investigations are necessary.

Arthritic conditions

Arthritis affects 2% of the population[256]. Rheumatoid arthritis affecting the feet requires specialist referral. Early diagnosis is assisted by eliciting pain on transverse tarsal pressure. The 'daylight' sign is due to swelling around the metatarsal–phalangeal joints which forces the metatarsal heads apart so that daylight may be seen between individual toes. The seronegative arthritides (ankylosing spondylitis, Reiter's disease, psoriatic arthritides) can all affect the feet, especially the heel. In gout, 75% of cases present with big toe problems. In England, a high proportion are diagnosed as cellulitis and treated with penicillin. It is well to be conscious of this condition because, if correctly diagnosed, it is treatable.

6
Anatomical Illustrations

THE MOBILE SEGMENT

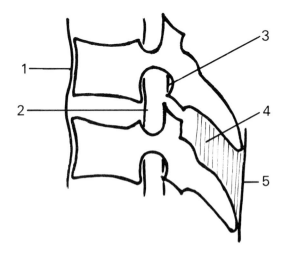

1. Anterior longitudinal ligament
2. Posterior longitudinal ligament
3. Ligamentum flavum
4. Interspinous ligament
5. Supraspinous ligament

CERVICAL LIGAMENTS – C0–1–2 – SAGITTAL VIEW

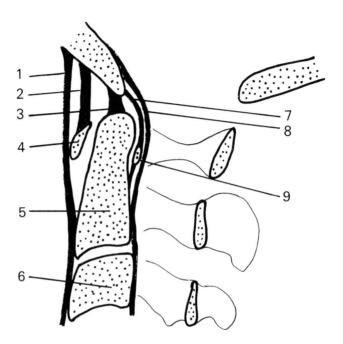

1. Anterior longitudinal ligament
2. Anterior occipitoatlantal membrane
3. Apical ligament
4. Anterior arch of atlas
5. Odontoid process
6. Vertebral body – C3
7. Occipitotransverse ligament
8. Median occipitoatlantal ligament – posterior longitudinal
9. Transverse ligament

THE COURSE OF THE VERTEBRAL ARTERY

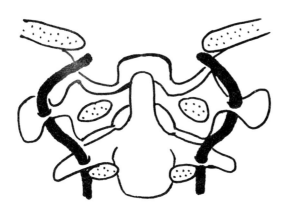

7
Diagnostic Techniques

APPARENT DIFFERENCE IN LEG LENGTH

There is no clear evidence as to the significance of differences in leg length in the aetiology of spinal symptoms. It is, however, in some cases of clinical importance.

A clinically acceptable method of assessment is to stand the patient on a level floor, with his toes slightly turned in and his knees straight, the examiner crouching behind him and placing his thumbs over the sacro-iliac dimples and his forefingers along the crests of the ilia. 'Sighting' along the lines so defined against any horizontal feature at once reveals any tilt of significance. Any doubt may be resolved by 'chocking up' the leg thought to be the shorter on a platform of known thickness and resighting.

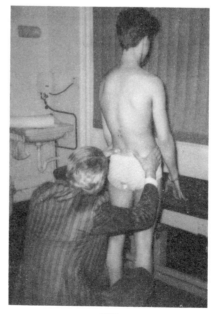

A minor refinement is the employment of a 10 cm grid against which to view the patient.

This method is very much more accurate than the use of a tape measure, especially in obese patients, in whom the anterior superior iliac spine is often impalpable.

SKIN DRAG

This test seeks to identify areas of skin in which there is an increase of resistance to movement of the examiner's finger over the skin on one side in comparison with the other.

The examination is conducted with the patient standing, the examiner running his index fingers down the patient's back, equidistant from the midline by approximately 2 cm with a light stroking touch, from occiput to buttocks. Sometimes the patient is able to feel a difference between the two sides.

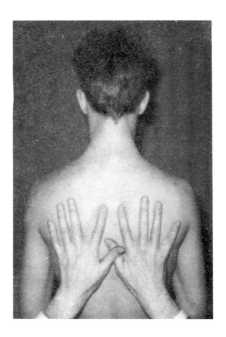

POSTERIOR SKIN ROLLING

This test seeks to reveal areas of tenderness of skin or subcutaneous tissue. It may be conducted with the patient standing, sitting or prone.

The examiner raises a fold of skin between forefingers and thumbs, pinching lightly and rolling the skinfold in the same distribution as for testing skin drag, from occiput to buttocks, asking the patient to advise him of any difference in discomfort between the two sides.

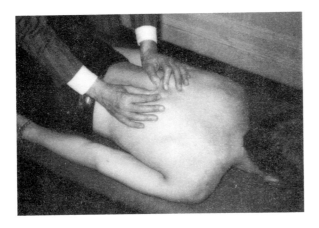

ANTERIOR SKIN ROLLING

Like posterior skin rolling, this test seeks to reveal areas of tenderness of skin or subcutaneous tissues. It must be emphasized that this is to be sought as widely anteriorly as it is posteriorly, a fact not generally appreciated in Britain, as we illustrate with the 'eyebrow' test of Maigne, the facial test and the trunk test.

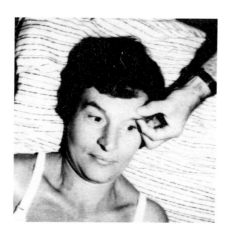 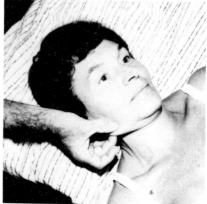

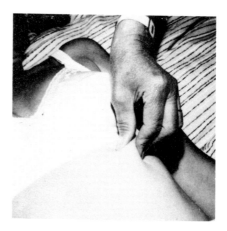

LATERAL SPINOUS PROCESS PRESSURE TEST

This test seeks to elicit pain on rotating a vertebra in one direction or the other. It may be conducted with the patient sitting or prone.

The examiner asks the patient to tell him if he experiences pain on pressure at any level or in either direction. He presses firmly and medially with his thumb against each spinous process from C7 to L5, both to the left and to the right.

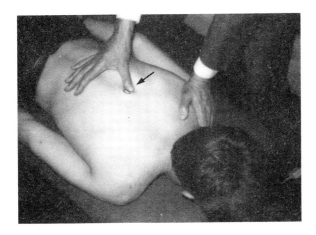

SPRINGING

This test seeks to elicit pain on applying a sagittal force to the spinous process of a vertebra. It is conducted with the patient prone.

The examiner places the ulnar border of either hand on each spinous process in turn, from C7 to L5, leans firmly upon it, reinforcing the pressure with the other hand, and gently springs the vertebra by a light, vertical thrust at each level.

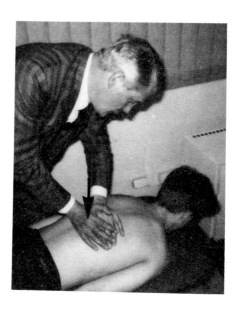

MUSCLE TONE TEST

This test seeks to identify areas in which there is increased muscle tone (or undue flaccidity) in the paravertebral musculature. It is best conducted supine for the cervical muscles, prone for the thoracic and lumbar muscles.

The examiner palpates transversely to the general direction of the muscle fibres, noting differences at different levels and between the two sides.

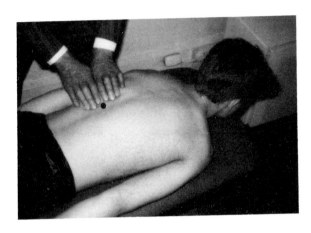

ZYGOAPOPHYSEAL TENDERNESS

This test seeks to reveal any tenderness there may be of the zygo-apophyseal posterior joint capsules and adjacent structures, in an attempt to define the site of the problem. As with the test for muscle tone, it is best conducted with the patient supine for the cervical spine, but prone for thoracic and lumbar joints.

The examiner asks the patient to report tenderness at any site. He presses deeply through the overlying tissues onto the posterior aspect of each zygoapophyseal joint in turn, finding these approximately one (patient's) finger's breadth lateral to the spinous processes. It must be remembered that in the thoracic spine the spinous processes are oblique, so as to bring each into line with the apophyseal joint one segment caudal to it.

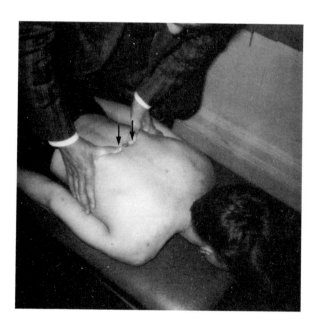

THE BELLPUSH SIGN OF MAIGNE

This sign is elicited by deep palpation of the anterolateral aspects of the cervical spine. A positive response is localized tenderness, with or without pain referred posteriorly or anteriorly.

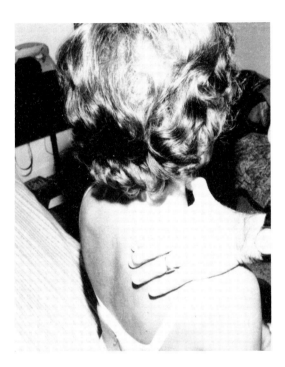

8
Manipulative Techniques

There are many techniques, of which we deliberately present relatively few. The reason for this is that, in practice, experienced manipulators commonly use but a small selection, because they find these particularly effective. This is in tune with the evidence as to the articular neurology presented in Chapter 1 on General Considerations.

We therefore present a 'Rosette' system, in the style of the *Guide Michelin*, in order to indicate the frequency with which we use the various techniques shown.

UPPER CERVICAL ROTATION – SUPINE ★★★

Positioning

Adjust the couch level to your umbilicus: Lie the patient supine, with her head supported in a position of comfort. Stand to the left of her head and, lying your right forearm beside her right ear, roll her head on to your forearm, your fingers just cupping her chin. Place the midshaft of the proximal phalanx of your left index finger over the left articular pillar at the level you wish to manipulate, your left thumb pointing anteriorly. To manipulate the upper segments, bend the neck over the fulcrum of your left index finger, and take up the slack in both right rotation and extension, maintaining close contact between the patient's head and your chest.

Manipulation

The final thrust is an accentuation of the positioning, your left index finger increasing extension by thrusting towards your right palm. This movement must be performed on a relaxed patient.

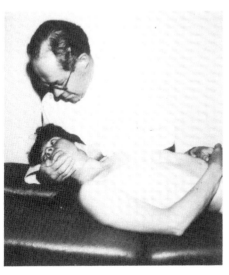
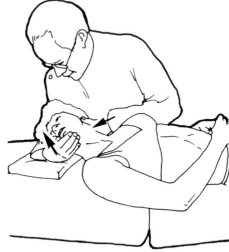

LOWER CERVICAL ROTATION – SUPINE ★★

Adjust the couch level to your umbilicus.

Positioning

To manipulate the lower segments, position the patient as for the upper segments, rotating to the right, and extending the neck. Place the midshaft of the proximal phalanx of your left index finger over the left articular pillar at the level you wish to manipulate, your left thumb pointing anteriorly. Then bend the neck towards the patient's chest, over the fulcrum of your left index finger. Take up the slack, maintaining close contact between her head and your chest.

Manipulation

The final thrust is an accentuation of the positioning, as in the upper segment manoeuvre, again with your left index finger thrusting towards your right palm. The movement must be rapid and of short amplitude.

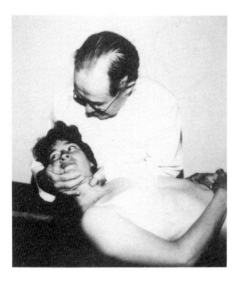
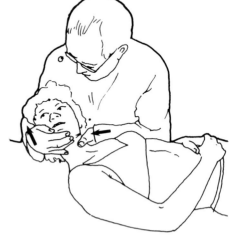

UPPER CERVICAL ROTATION IN TRACTION – SITTING 1   ★★

Positioning

Seat the patient comfortably on a chair. Stand immediately behind the patient. Reaching over her right shoulder with your right arm, ask the patient to turn her head to the left and drop the right side of her head on to your right wrist. The fingers of your right hand cup her chin. Place the heel of your left hand over the patient's left occiput, the thumb along the occipital ridge, the fingers extending over the parietal bone.

Manipulation

Ensure the patient is relaxed, then take up the slack in left rotation, flexion and right side-bending, at the same time exerting quite a strong vertical traction with the right forearm, bringing her head into close contact with your chest. The final thrust is a rapid, short-amplitude accentuation of the positioning.

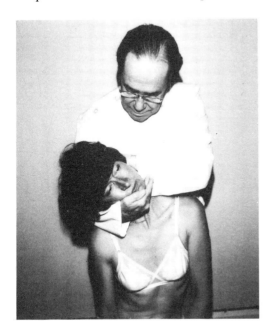
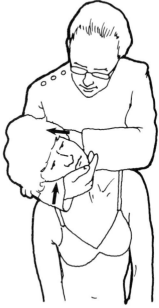

UPPER CERVICAL ROTATION IN TRACTION – SITTING 2 ★★★

Positioning

Seat the patient comfortably on a chair. Stand immediately behind him. Reaching over his left shoulder with your left arm, ask him to turn his head fully to the left and to drop the right side of his face onto your hand and wrist. Place the heel of your right hand over his left occiput.

Manipulation

Take up the slack and exert strong vertical traction with your left hand and forearm, bringing his head into close contact with your chest and pressing firmly downwards and forwards with your right hand. The final thrust is a rapid, short-amplitude accentuation of the positioning.

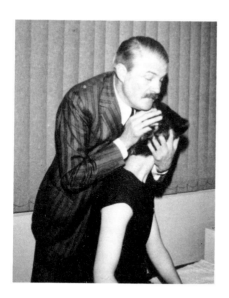 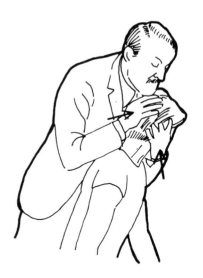

LOWER CERVICAL ROTATION – SITTING ★★★

Positioning

Seat the patient sideways on a chair. Stand immediately behind her and place your left foot on the seat of the chair, adjacent to her left hip. Drape the patient's left arm over your left thigh and apply your right thumb to the right side of her 7th cervical spinous process. Ask the patient to lean her head to the right and rotate left. Place your left palm on her left forehead and take up the slack in left rotation, extension and right side-bending, ensuring her head is closely applied to your chest.

Manipulation

The final thrust is a rapid, short-amplitude accentuation of the positioning. The patient must be relaxed at the moment of thrust.

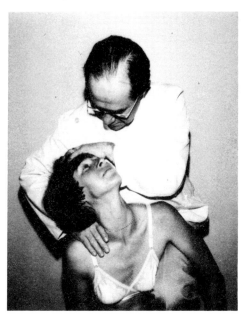
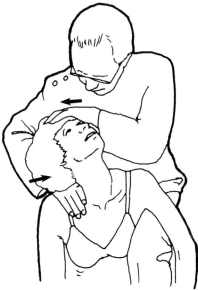

CERVICAL SIDE-BENDING   ★

Positioning

Adjust the couch to the level of your crutch. Lie the patient on his left side, with his head well clear of the end of the couch and supported on your left wrist and forearm, your left hand cupping his chin. Apply the proximal phalanx of your right index finger over the right transverse process at the required level.

Manipulation

Take up the slack, bringing the patient into maximal side-bending to the right over the fulcrum of your down-thrusting right index finger. The manipulation is a rapid, short-amplitude accentuation of the positioning.

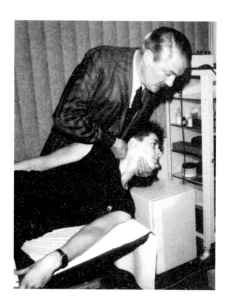
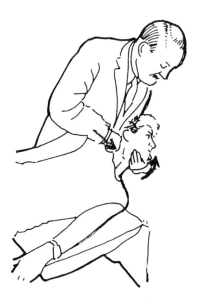

PRONE CERVICAL ROTATION – CHIN PIVOT ★

Positioning

Adjust the couch level to your mid-thigh. Lie the patient prone, his neck extended sufficient to bring his chin onto the couch. Side-bend his head to the right. Apply your right thumb to the left lateral aspect of his 7th cervical spinous process. Place your left hand over the patient's right ear, fingers towards his chin, the heel of your hand over the parietal region. Opposing pressure between your right thumb and left hand will produce right rotation, while retaining some extension, as the patient pivots on his chin.

Manipulation

Taking up the slack, the manipulation is a rapid, short-amplitude accentuation of the positioning.

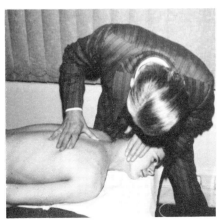
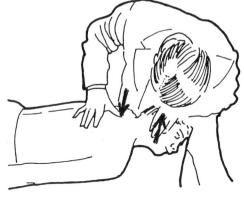

LOWER CERVICAL ROTATION – PRONE ★

Positioning

Adjust the couch level to your mid-thigh. Lie the patient prone, his head well clear of the end of the couch. Support his right cheek with your left hand and side-bend and rotate his head to the left. Apply your right thumb to the lateral aspect of his 7th cervical spinous process.

Manipulation

Taking up the slack, this is a rapid, short-amplitude thrust by your right thumb, while accentuating the rotation with your left hand.

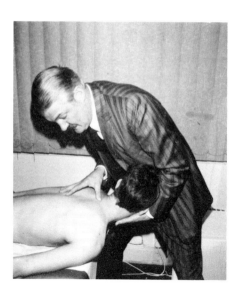
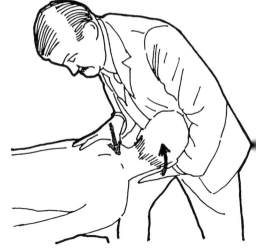

STERNAL THRUST – STANDING ★★★

Positioning

Ask the patient to stand relaxed. Standing behind her, ask her to link her fingers behind her neck, pass your forearms anterior to her upper arms, so as to clasp her wrists with your hands. Fold the patient's elbows forwards and flex her neck, applying your sternum to her back, at the level you wish to manipulate. By flexing your arms at the elbow pull the patient towards your chest.

Manipulation

When the slack is taken up, apply a thrust rapidly and with restraint, by accentuation of the positioning, the thrust being applied by your sternum.

Positioning: a modification for tall patients

To position your sternum, ask the patient to keep her feet still and relax, reassure her that you will not drop her, and pull her over backwards, moving your feet back at the same time, until such time as the desired level of her thoracic spine is in contact with your sternum. You may find it 'safer' to move back against a wall or sturdy piece of furniture.

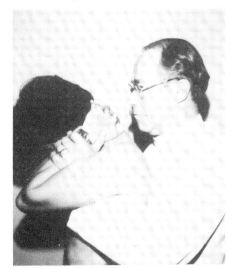 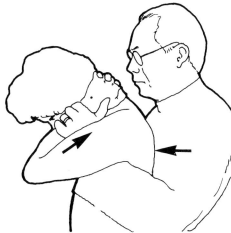

STERNAL THRUST – SITTING ★★

Positioning

Sit the patient on a stool or couch, of a height to put her head on a level with your own. Standing behind her, ask her to link her fingers behind her neck, pass your forearms anterior to her upper arms, and clasp her wrists with your hands. Fold the patient's elbows forwards and flex her neck, applying your sternum to her back, at the level you wish to manipulate. By flexing your elbows pull her towards your chest.

Manipulation

When the slack is taken up, apply a thrust rapidly and with restraint, by accentuation of the positioning, pulling backwards so as to introduce an element of traction into the manoeuvre.

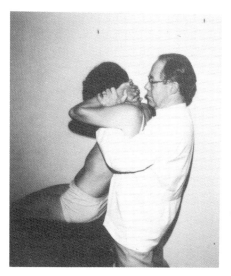
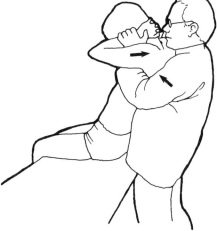

STERNAL THRUST – SUPINE ★★

Positioning

The patient lies supine, fingers linked behind her neck, elbows together. Stand to her right and, rolling her towards you, place your
right thenar eminence over the left transverse process, your hand
crossing the midline, all fingers being on the right of her spinous
process of choice. Roll her back on to your right hand, clasping her
elbows with your left hand, and flex her cervicothoracic spine to the
required degree and apply your sternum closely over your left hand
and her forearms.

Manipulation

Take up the slack, and make a rapid, short manipulative thrust with
your sternum vertically towards your right thenar eminence.

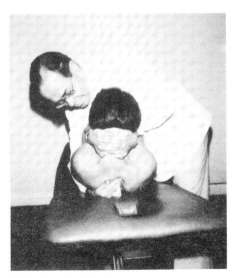
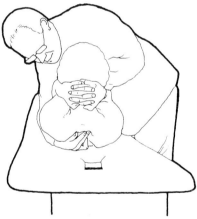

Modification

This technique may be modified for lower thoracic levels by increasing the degree of cervicothoracic flexion.

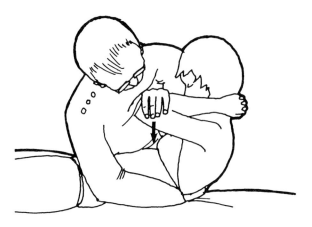

CROSSED PISIFORM THRUST – 1 ★★

Positioning

Lie the patient prone. Select the level at which manipulation is desired, remembering that the tips of the thoracic spinous processes overlap the vertebra below. Stand on the patient's left, and place your left pisiform bone over her left 5th transverse process, the fingers and thumb pointing to your right. Place your right pisiform bone over her right 4th transverse process, the fingers and thumb pointing to your left.

Manipulation

Bending well over the patient, lean vertically downwards, both elbows slightly flexed, taking up the slack. Ask her to inhale deeply and then exhale. At the end of exhalation increase the downward force by a sharp, controlled thrust, achieved by extending both elbows simultaneously.

For the sake of description, this manoeuvre is in part aimed at rotating the 4th thoracic vertebra anticlockwise on the 5th.

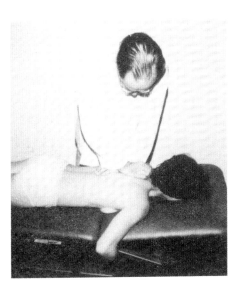
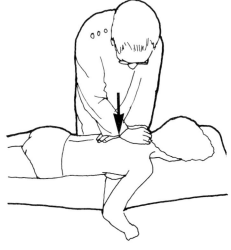

CROSSED PISIFORM THRUST – 2   ★★

Positioning

This manoeuvre must be modified for manipulation at lower levels, the pressure of your pisiform bones being applied obliquely in a cephalic direction, progressively more so the lower the manipulation.

Manipulation

The thrust is a rapid, controlled accentuation of the positioning. The patient must be relaxed, and she should be forewarned that this procedure may be unpleasant.

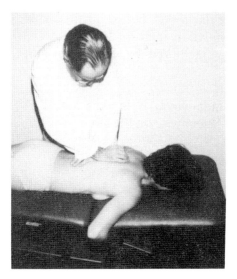 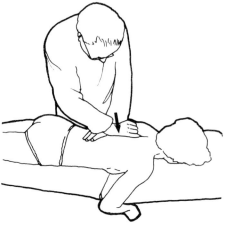

KNEE IN BACK ★

Positioning

Sit the patient on a stool or couch just higher than your patellae. Standing behind her, ask her to link her fingers behind her neck, pass your forearms anterior to her upper arms and clasp her wrists with your hands. Place either foot on the couch behind her buttocks and apply your knee over the transverse process you wish to move, adjusting the height of your knee by extension or flexion of your ankle. Fold the patient's elbows forward and flex her neck, bringing her into firm contact with your knee, taking up the slack by flexing your elbows.

Manipulation

When the slack has been taken up, apply a thrust rapidly and with restraint, by accentuation of the positioning, the thrust being applied by your knee.

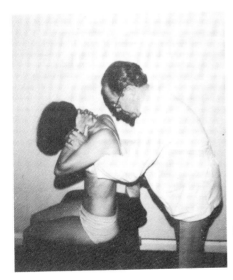
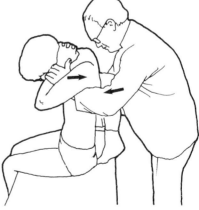

SPINOUS PROCESS ROTATION ★

Positioning

Adjust the height of the couch to just above your patellae. Lie the patient prone. Standing on either side of the couch, place your thumbs against the lateral aspects of two neighbouring spinous processes, one on either side.

Manipulation

This is achieved by opposing thrusts between your two thumbs, each directed towards the midline, thereby attempting a rotation concentrated at the level required. It is, in effect, a bilateral accentuation of the lateral spinous process pressure test (see Chapter 7), with the emphasis of the thrust in the pain-free direction.

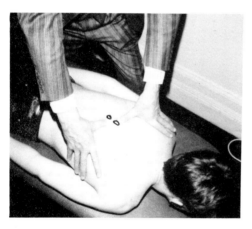 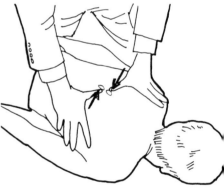

THORACIC ROTATION – SITTING ★

Positioning

Adjust the couch level to just above your patellae. Sit the patient on the couch, legs apart, her hands clasped behind her neck. Pass your right hand anterior to her right upper arm and bring it to overlie her hands. Place your left thumb on the left lateral aspect of the spinous process at the level to be manipulated. Rotate her trunk to the right and bring her into marked flexion, leaning your chest on her right scapular region.

Manipulation

Taking up the slack, this is a rapid, short-amplitude thrust with your left thumb simultaneous to accentuation of rotation and flexion with your right arm and chest.

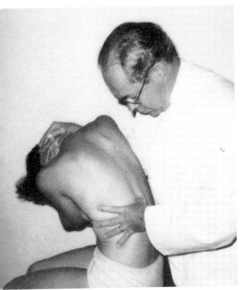
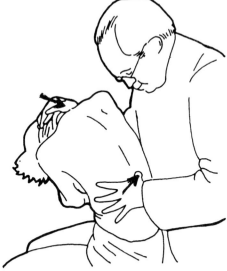

LUMBAR ROTATION   ★★★★

Positioning

Lie the patient on her right side, her head lying on her right hand. Stand in front of her. Rotate her trunk to the left by placing your left forearm in the sulcus between her left shoulder and chest. Flex her left knee and hip, and place your right forearm over her left upper buttock. With fingers of both hands palpate the spinous processes above and below the level you wish to move. Use both forearms to increase rotation, monitoring the resultant movement with your finger tips.

Manipulation

Taking up the slack, the manipulation is executed by a sharp increase of rotatory pressure by both forearms, as illustrated.

This technique may be modified for higher levels by pulling her right shoulder forwards and downwards, thereby increasing thoracolumbar flexion.

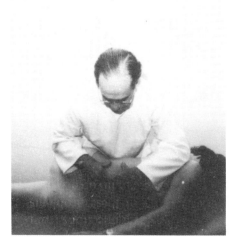
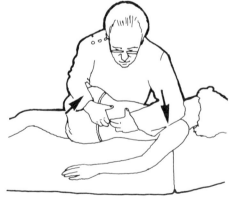

LUMBOSACRAL – PRONE 1 ★★

Positioning

Lie the patient prone. Stand on the patient's left side (for a right-sided problem). Place the heel of your left hand over her right sacro-iliac joint, bearing down firmly. With your right hand grasp the anterior aspect of her right thigh, just above the knee, hyper-extending her right hip, taking up the slack.

Manipulation

Thrust vertically downwards with your left hand, while accentuating hyperextension of her right hip with your right hand.

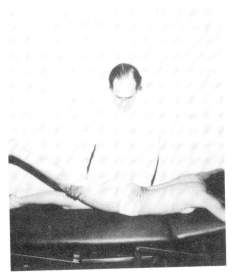
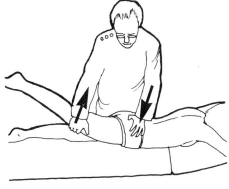

LUMBAR ROTATION – SITTING   ★

Positioning

Adjust the couch level to just above your patellae. Sit the patient on the couch, legs apart, his hands clasped behind his neck. Pass your right hand anterior to his right upper arm and bring it to overlie his hands. Place your left thumb on the left lateral aspect of the spinous process at the level to be manipulated. Rotate his trunk to the right and bring him into flexion, leaning your chest on his right scapular area.

Manipulation

Taking up the slack, this is a rapid, short-amplitude thrust with your left thumb simultaneous to accentuation of rotation and flexion with your right arm and chest.

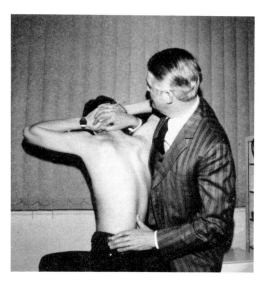
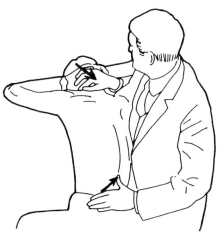

LUMBAR EXTENSION – SITTING ★

Positioning

Adjust the couch level to just above your patellae. Sit the patient on the couch, hands clasped behind his neck. Place either knee at the level selected for manipulation, in the midline, separated from the patient by a small, firm cushion. This will necessitate resting your foot on a platform of suitable height. Pass both your hands anterior to his upper arms and clasp his forearms just above his wrists.

Manipulation

Extend his back over the fulcrum of your knee until the slack is taken up. The manipulative thrust is a rapid, short-amplitude accentuation of the positioning.

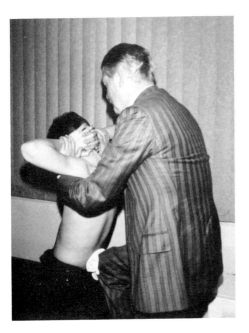
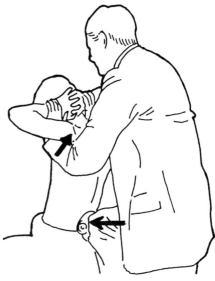

LUMBOSACRAL FORWARD THRUST ★

Positioning

Adjust couch level to just above your patellae. Lie the patient on his right side at the edge of the couch, his left leg hanging over the edge of the couch. Grasp his left leg between your thighs, so as to provide stability. Place the heel of either hand over his left posterior superior iliac spine, reinforcing the downward pressure with your other hand.

Manipulation

This is a rapid, short-amplitude vertical thrust.

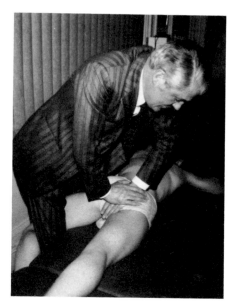
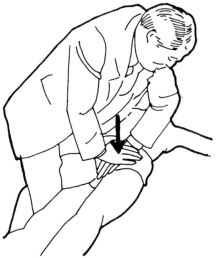

LUMBOSACRAL LONGITUDINAL THRUST

Positioning

Adjust couch level to your mid-thigh. Lie the patient on her right side near the edge of the couch, her left leg dangling over the side. Grasp her left leg between your thighs, so as to provide greater stability. Place your left hand on her left shoulder, your right hand on her left iliac crest, exerting firm pressure down the axes of each forearm.

Manipulation

Take up the slack; the manipulation is a rapid, short-amplitude thrust with both hands.

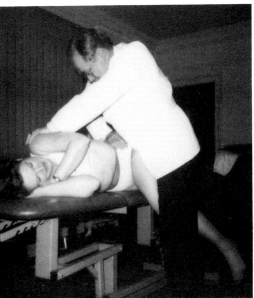
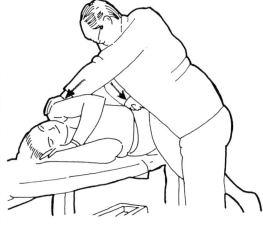

LUMBOSACRAL – PRONE 2 ★

Positioning

Adjust the height of the couch to just above your patellae. Lie the patient prone, then ask her to rear up onto her elbows, her upper arms vertical. Stand on her left side and push your left knee under her rib cage, just behind her left upper arm. Place the heel of your right hand over her right sacro-iliac joint and pass your left arm over her right shoulder, reaching round with your left hand over her right lower ribs. Rotate her to the right by rolling her trunk up your left thigh, sufficient to lift her right anterior superior iliac spine off the couch.

Manipulation

Taking up the slack, the manipulation is executed by a sharp downward thrust with your right hand.

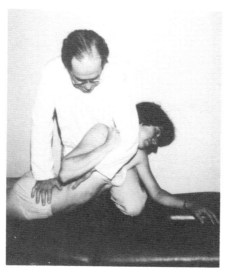
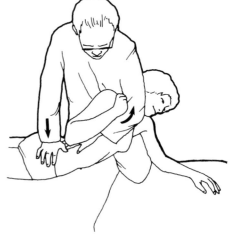

MILLION DOLLAR ROLL

This technique is included as being of historical interest. It is still widely used, but we do not recommend it because it is over-forceful, uncontrolled and entirely non-specific.

Positioning

Adjust the height of the couch to just above your patellae. Lie the patient on her right side and stand in front of her. Bring her close to the edge of the couch, with her head lying on her right hand. Rotate her trunk to the left, by pushing her left shoulder away with your left hand, at the same time flexing her left hip and knee, tucking her left toes behind her right knee. Increase rotation by pressing her left shoulder back, your right hand pushing her left knee downwards.

Manipulation

Taking up the slack, the manipulation is executed by a sharp and simultaneous increase in pressure by both hands. This technique may be modified for higher levels by pulling her right shoulder downwards and forwards, thereby increasing thoracolumbar flexion.

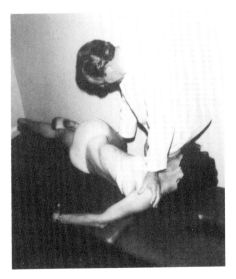
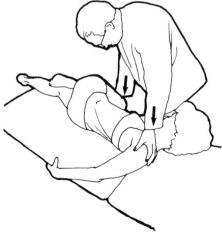

9
Injections

OCCIPITAL INJECTIONS

General

These may be of value in occipitovertebral headache believed to originate in the cervical spine. Some appear to be related to the greater occipital nerve of Arnold, others to the attachment tissues of the long posterior muscles of the neck.

Materials

The materials used are local anaesthetic and steroid, the choice of which offers wide variation and is a matter of individual preference. The volume injected will depend upon how wide an infiltration is desired – usually between 3 ml and 6 ml.

Technique

Seek the sites of maximum tenderness along the superior occipital line. Using a 25SWG needle, penetrate until the needle tip reaches bone, withdraw minimally and inject widely in the vicinity.

CERVICAL APOPHYSEAL INJECTIONS

General

Owing to the unpredictably variable course of the vertebral artery, these injections should be limited to levels below C2. With this exclusion they remain a most valuable form of therapy.

Materials

As for the occipital injections.

Technique

Tell the patient to look slightly up and forwards and to hold still: the extension of his neck ensures superimposition of the cervical laminae. It is important to eliminate any side-bending or rotation. Using a 21SWG 1½-inch needle, insert horizontally at the selected level, one finger's breadth lateral to the midline, until the needle point reaches bone. This is of vital importance as a safety measure. Withdraw the plunger slightly to ensure that there is no blood, then inject about 2 ml of the mixture, withdraw partially and inject in the vicinity of the joints above and below, as the innervation of all apophyseal joints must involve *at least three levels*.

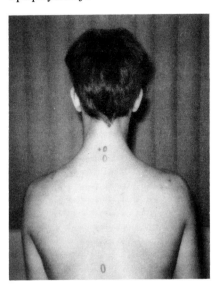 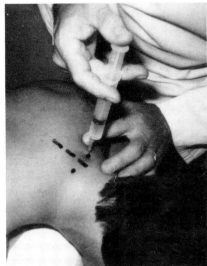

THORACIC APOPHYSEAL JOINT INJECTIONS

Materials

As for the cervical injections.

Technique

Lie the patient prone. Remember that in a muscular or obese patient, the zygoapophyseal joint may be 4–5 cm deep from the skin. Therefore, use a 21SWG needle of adequate length. Insert the needle vertically at the selected level, one finger's breadth from the midline, until the needle point reaches bone, remembering that the tip of the spinous process in the thoracic spine is level with the apophyseal joint of the segment immediately caudal to the spinous process. Proceed otherwise as for the cervical injection.

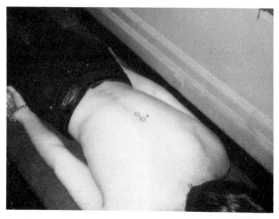

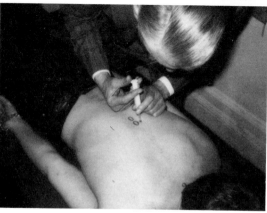

LUMBAR APOPHYSEAL INJECTIONS

Materials

As for the thoracic apophyseal joint injections.

Technique

Lie the patient prone. Because the zygoapophyseal joint in the adult lumbar spine is some 5 cm deep from the skin, it is necessary to use a needle of adequate length. Insert the needle vertically at the selected level, one finger's breadth from the midline beside the spinous process, until the needle point reaches bone, and proceed otherwise as described for the thoracic spine technique.

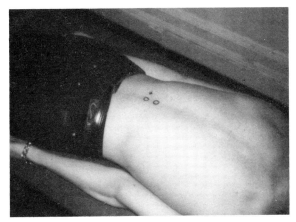

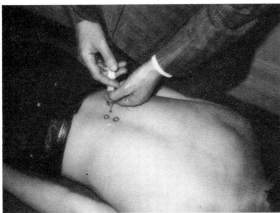

CAUDAL EPIDURAL ANAESTHESIA

General

This is a simple, safe technique, suitable for use in the surgery. The dangers of the procedure are three: local sepsis, anaphylactoid reaction to the local anaesthetic and a volume injected in excess of 50 ml. The volume most commonly employed is between 10 ml and 20 ml. Opinions differ regarding the materials used, which suggests that there is no clear advantage of one over another. Most commonly a mixture of anaesthetic and steroid is used. The lumbar approach is similar to that used in lumbar puncture. It is contraindicated in general practice because the technical difficulties and the risks are significant.

Technique

Lie the patient prone. Identify the sacral hiatus by palpation of the cornua of the sacrum, the hiatus lying between these landmarks. The hiatus will be impalpable in very obese patients, in which case the procedure is abandoned. Using a 21SWG 1½-inch or 2-inch needle, insert it in the midline, perpendicular to the skin, so as to just penetrate the fibrous tissue roof of the sacral cavity. Once the tip of

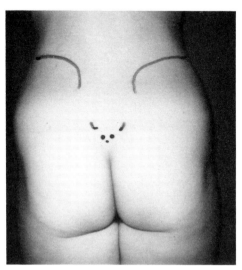 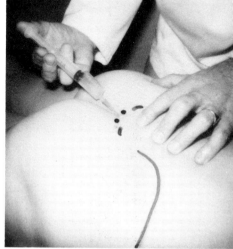

the needle is perceived to have penetrated this structure, alter the angle of the needle so as to point up the sacrum, as far as this angle may be judged. Then insert about a further $\frac{3}{4}$-1 inch, withdraw the plunger, so as to ascertain whether you have entered a blood vessel; if blood is found, withdraw the needle a little and re-test; if no blood is found, inject the chosen solution *slowly*. The length of time a patient is kept recumbent following this procedure varies widely from clinician to clinician, with no clear indication of the ideal period.

If the patient complains of pain, the injection should be given more slowly than if she does not. Several minutes must be allowed.

10
Back Exercises

LYING EXERCISE

Lie on your back, with your arms crossed over your chest. Keeping your knees straight, lift both legs off the couch, at the same time lifting your head and shoulders. Hold this position for about 10 seconds, rest for 5 seconds and repeat as directed. You *must* repeat this exercise night and morning, starting with four repetitions, adding two each week, to a maximum of 20, and continuing for life.

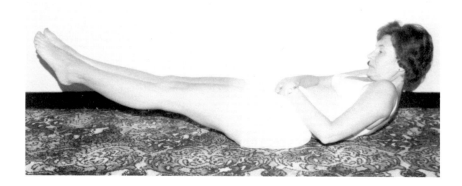

STANDING EXERCISE

Stand with your feet about 18 inches (50 cm) apart, your toes slightly turned inwards. Turn the palms of your hands to the front, then twist them round, forcing your thumbs backwards, at the same time tightening the muscles of your buttocks. Hold this position for about 10 seconds, relax for 5 seconds and repeat as directed. As with the lying exercise, you *must* repeat this night and morning, starting with four repetitions, adding two each week, to a maximum of 20, and continuing for life.

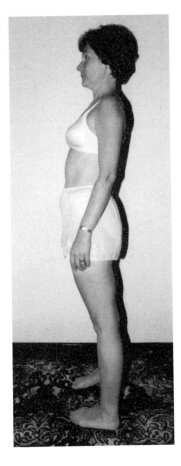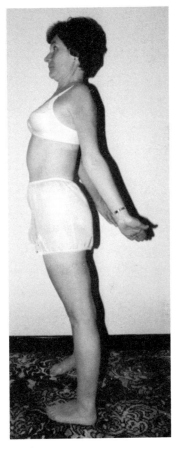

11
Domiciliary Traction

CERVICAL AUTOSUSPENSION

The simplest autosuspension unit comprises a steel spreader bar, strong but light in weight, suspended from a suitable hook in the patient's home. This latter must be securely fixed, in particular not to a banister.

The head harness consists of two webbing pieces, one for the chin, the other for the occiput, freely running on two nylon cords.

The apparatus is shown below, from which it will be seen that traction is obtained by the patient bending her knees – she may take her feet off the floor, but this is usually rather uncomfortable.

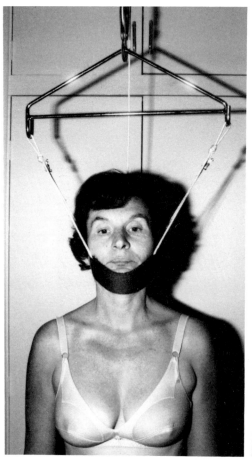
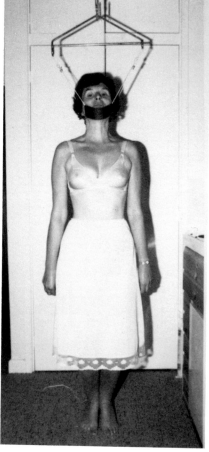

LUMBAR AUTOSUSPENSION

This is the counterpart of the cervical autosuspension unit.

The spreader bar, wider than that for cervical traction and fitted with a hook at either end, takes a swivel bar on either hook, using the second hole from the outer end. The head harness, identical to that used in the cervical unit, is slung between the innermost holes of the two swivel bars, the axillary loops being hung from the outer holes on each side. The whole is suspended as described, the axillary loops adjusted so as to leave the swivel bars roughly horizontal with the patient standing comfortably.

Traction is applied by the patient bending her knees – she may take her feet off the floor in perfect safety, if she so wishes.

Apparatus is shown below.

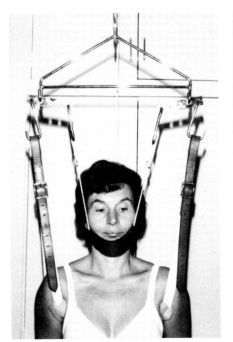 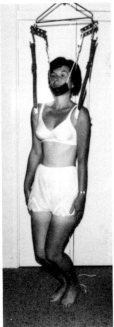

References

1 Wall, P.D. (1978). The gate control theory of pain mechanisms: a re-examination and restatement. *Brain*, **101**, 1

2 Stoddard, A. (1983). *A Manual of Osteopathic Practice*. 2nd Edn. (London: Hutchinson Medical)

3 Wyke, B.D. (1970). The neurological basis of thoracic spinal pain. *Rheum. Phys. Med.*, **10**, 356

4 Wyke, B.D. (1983). Presentation at *7th International Congress of FIMM*, Zürich

5 Haldeman, S. (1982). Presentation at *Colt Symposium*

6 Dove, C. (1982). Presentation at *Colt Symposium*

7 Hilton, R.C. (1980). In Jayson, M. (ed.) *The Lumbar Spine and Back Pain*. 2nd Edn. (Tunbridge Wells: Pitman Medical)

8 Moll, J. and Wright, V. (1980). In Jayson, M. (ed.) *The Lumbar Spine and Back Pain*. 2nd Edn. (Tunbridge Wells: Pitman Medical)

9 Anderson, J.A.D. (1976). In Jayson, M. (ed.) *The Lumbar Spine and Back Pain*. (Tunbridge Wells: Pitman Medical)

10 Hay, M.C. (1974). The incidence of low back pain in Busselton. In Twomey, L.T. (ed.) *Symposium: Low Back Pain*. (Perth: Western Australia Institute of Technology)

11 Cust, G., Pearson, J.C.G. and Mair, A. (1972). The prevalence of low back pain in nurses. *Int. Nurs. Rev.*, **19**, 169-79

12 Hult, L. (1954). Cervical, dorsal, and lumbar spinal syndromes. *Acta Orthop. Scand.* (Suppl.), 17

13 Bergquist-Ullman, M. and Larsson, U. (1977). Acute low back pain in industry. *Acta Orthop. Scand.* (Suppl.), **170**

14 Magora, A. (1972). Investigation of the relation between low back pain and occupation. 3. Physical requirements: Sitting, standing and weight lifting. *Ind. Med. Surg*, **41**, 5-9

15 Kelsey, J.L. and Hardy, R.J. (1975). Driving of motor vehicles as a risk factor for acute herniated lumbar intervertebral disc. *Am. J. Epidemiol.*, **102**, 63-73

16 Andersson, G.B.J. (1982). Presentation at *Colt Symposium*

17 Troup, J.D.G., Roantree, W.B. and Archibald, R.M. (1970). Survey of cases of lumbar spinal disability. A methodological study. *Med. Officers' Broadsheet, National Coal Board*

18 Chaffin, D.B. and Park, K.S. (1973). A longitudinal study of low back pain as associated with occupational weight lifting factors. *Am. Ind. Hyg. Assoc. J.*, **34**, 513-25

19 Berkson, M., Schultz, A., Nachemson, A. and Andersson, G.B.J. (1977). Voluntary strengths of male adults with acute low back syndromes. *Clin. Orthop.*, **129**, 84-95

20 Dupuis, H. and Christ, W. (1972). Untersuchung der Möglichkeit von Gesundheits-schädigungen im Bereich der Wirbelsäule bei Schlepperfahrern. (Max Plank Institute, Bad Kreuznach, Heft A72/2)

21 Fitzgerald, H.G. and Crotty, J. (1972). The incidence of backache among aircrew and groundcrew in the RAF. FPRC/1313

22 Taylor, D.G. (1976). The costs of arthritis and the benefits of joint replacement surgery. *Proc. R. Soc. Med.*, **192**, 145–55

23 Andersson, G.B.J. (1981). Epidemiologic aspects on low back pain in industry. *Spine*, **6**, 53–60

24 Brown, J.R. (1973). Lifting as an industrial hazard. *Am. Ind. Hyg. Assoc. J.*, **34**, 292

25 O'Brien, J. (1984). In Melzack, R. and Wall, P.D. (eds.) *A Textbook of Pain*

26 Magora, A. (1970). Investigation of the relation between low back pain and occupation. 2. Work history. *Ind. Med. Surg.*, **39**, 504–10

27 Nachemson, A.L. (1969). Back problems in childhood and adolescence. *Lakartidningen*, **65**, 2831–43 (In Swedish)

28 Tauber, J. (1970). An unorthodox look at backaches. *J. Occup. Med.*, **12**, 128–30

29 Ikata, T. (1965). Statistical and dynamic studies of lesions due to overloading on the spine. *Shikoku Acta Med.*, **40**, 262–86

30 Farfan, H.F. (1973). *Mechanical Disorders of the Low Back*. (Philadelphia: Lea & Febiger)

31 Cady, L.D., Bischoff, D.P., O'Connell, E.R., Thomas, T.C. and Allan, J.H. (1979). Strengths and fitness and subsequent back injuries in firefighters. *J. Occup. Med.*, **21**, 269–72

32 Kellgren, J.H. (1939). On the distribution of pain arising from deep somatic structures with charts of segmental pain areas. *Clin. Sci.*, **4**, 35

33 Frykholm, R. (1971). The clinical picture. In Hirsch, C. and Zotterman, Y. (eds.) *Cervical Pain*. p. 5. (Oxford: Pergamon)

34 Cloward, R.B. (1959). Cervical diskography. *Ann. Surg.*, **150**, 1052

35 Holt, E.P. (1964) Fallacy of cervical discography: report of 50 cases in normal subjects. *J. Am. Med. Assoc.*, **188**, 799

36 Klafta, L.A. and Collis, J.S. (1969). The diagnostic inaccuracy of the pain response in cervical discography. *Clev. Clin. Q.*, **36**, 35

37 Kirk, E.J. and Denny-Brown, D. (1970). Functional variations in dermatomes in the macaque monkey following dorsal root lesions. *J. Comp. Neurol.*, **139**, 307

38 Denny-Brown, D., Kirk, E.J. and Yanagisawa, N. (1973). The tract of Lissauer in relation to sensory transmission in the dorsal horn of the spinal cord in the macaque. *J. Comp. Neurol.*, **151**, 175

39 Last, R.J. (1978). *Anatomy, Regional and Applied*. 6th Edn. p. 27. (Edinburgh and London: Churchill Livingstone)

40 Mooney, V. and Robertson, J. (1976). The facet syndrome. *Clin. Orthop. Relat. Res.*, **115**, 149

41 Bourdillon, J.F. (1973). *Spinal Manipulation*. 2nd Edn. (London: Heinemann)

42 Keele, C.A. and Neil, E. (eds.) (1971). *Samson Wright's Applied Physiology*. 12th Edn. (London: Oxford UP)

43 Macnab, I. (1977) *Backache*. (Baltimore: Williams & Wilkins)

44 O'Brien, J.P. (1979). Anterior spinal tenderness in low back pain syndromes. *Spine*, **4**, 85

45 Grieve, G.P. (ed.) (1981). *Common Vertebral Joint Problems*. (Edinburgh and London: Churchill Livingstone)

46 Jayson, M.I.V. (ed.) (1976). *The Lumbar Spine and Back Pain*. (Tunbridge Wells: Pitman Medical)

REFERENCES

47 Froriep, A. (1843). *Ein Betrag zur Pathologie und Therapie des Rheumatismus.* (Weimar)

48 Gowers, W.R. (1904). Lumbago: its lessons and analogues. *Br. Med. J.*, **1**, 117

49 Copeman, W.S.C. and Ackerman, W.L. (1947). Oedema or herniations of fat lobules as a cause of lumbar and gluteal 'fibrositis'. *Arch. Intern. Med.*, **79**, 22

50 Travell, J., Rinzler, S.H. and Hermann, M. (1942). Pain and disability of the shoulder and arm. *J. Am. Med. Assoc.*, **120**, 417

51 Jayson, M.I.V. (ed.) (1980). *The Lumbar Spine and Back Pain.* 2nd Edn. (Tunbridge Wells: Pitman Medical)

52 Mooney, V., Cairns, D. and Robertson, J. (1976). A system for evaluating and treating chronic back disability. *West. J. Med.*, **124**, 370

53 Melzack, R., Stillwell, D.M. and Fox, E.J. (1977). Trigger points and acupuncture points for pain: correlations and implications. *Pain*, **3**, 23

54 Steindler, A. and Luck, J.V. (1938). Differential diagnosis of pain low in the back. *J. Am. Med. Assoc.*, **110**, 106

55 Simons, D.G. (1975). Muscle pain syndromes: Part I. *Am. J. Phys. Med.*, **54**, 289

56 Maigne, R. (1976). Un signe évocateur et inattendu de céphalée cervicale: la douleur au pince-roulé du sourcil. *Ann. Med. Phys.*, **4**, 416–34

57 International Association for the Study of Pain (1979). Pain terms: A list with definitions and notes on usage. IASP Subcommittee on Taxonomy. *Pain*, **6**, 249–52

58 Merskey, H. (1982). Presentation at *Colt Symposium*

59 Large, R.G. and Mullins, P.R. (1981). Illness behaviour profiles in chronic pain: the Auckland experience. *Pain*, **10**, 231–39

60 Pilowsky, I., Chapman, C.R. and Bonica, J.J. (1977). Pain, depression and illness behaviour in a pain clinic population. *Pain*, **4**, 183–92

61 Sternbach, R.A. (1974). *Pain Patients. Traits and Treatment.* (New York: Academic Press)

62 Woodforde, J.M. and Merskey, H. (1972). Personality traits of patients with chronic pain. *J. Psychosom. Res.*, **16**, 167–72

63 Engel, G.L. 'Psychogenic' pain and the pain-prone patient. *Am. J. Med.*, **26**, 899–918

64 Wyke, B.D. (1983). Presentation at *6th International Congress of FIMM*, Zurich

65 Grisel, P. (1930). Enucléation de l'atlas et torticollis nasopharyngien. *Presse Med.*, **38**, 50

66 von Gutmann, G. (1970). X-ray diagnosis of spinal dysfunction. *Man. Med.*, **4**, 73

67 Daneshmend, T.K. (1984). Acute brain stem stroke during neck manipulation. *Br. Med. J.*, **288**, 189

68 Jennett, W.B. (1956). A study of 25 cases of compression of the cauda equina by prolapsed intervertebral discs. *J. Neurol. Neurosurg. Psychiatry*, **19**, 109

69 Arnold, J. (1965). Fatal thrombosis of basilar artery after chiropractice. Quoted by Ford and Clark[79]

70 Attall, P. (1957). Accidents graves après manipulation intempestive par un chiropracteur. *Rev. Rheum.*, **24**, 652

71 Benassy, J. and Wolinetz, E. (1957). Quadriplégie après manoeuvre de chiropraxie. *Rev. Rheum.*, **24**, 555

72 Blaine, E.S. (1975). Chiropractic dislocation of atlas. *J. Am. Med. Assoc.*, **85**, 1356

73 Boshes, L.D. (1959). Vascular accidents associated with neck manipulation. *J. Am. Med. Assoc.*, **66**, 755

74 Bondin, G. and Barbizet, J. (1958). Des accidents nerveux de chiropraxie du rachis cervicale. *Rev. Practicien*, **8**, 2235

75 Dabbett, O., Freeman, D.G. and Weiss, D.G. (1970), Spinal meningeal haematoma, warfarin therapy and chiropractic adjustment. *J. Am. Med. Assoc.*, **214**, 2058

76 Degenering, P.W. (1961). Hazards of chiropractice. *Med. Klin.*, **56**, 1756

77 Deshayes, P. and Geoffroy, Y. (1962). Paralysie plexique supérieure, accident d'une manipulation vertébrale. *Rev. Rheum.*, **29**, 137

78 Easton, J.D. (1977), Chiropractic cerebral damage. (Lecture at *World Congress of Neurology*.) *Med. Post*, 22, November

79 Ford, F.R. and Clark, D. (1956). Thrombosis of basilar artery with softening of cerebellum due to manipulation of neck. *Bull. Johns Hopkins Hosp.*, **98**, 37

80 Green, D. and Joynt, R.J. (1959), Vascular accidents to the brain stem associated with neck manipulation. *J. Am. Med. Assoc.*, **182**, 255

81 Kreuger, B. (1980). Chiropractogenic stroke. *Med. Post*

82 Kreuger, B. and Okazaki, (1980). Vertebrobasilar infarction following chiropractic cervical manipulation. *Mayo Clin. Proc.*, **55**, 322

83 Lieure, J.A. (1953). Paraplégie du aux manoeuvres d'un chiropracteur. *Rev. Rheum.*, **20**, 708

84 Livingstone, M.C.P. (1971). Spinal manipulation causing injury. *Clin. Orthop.*, **81**, 82

85 Oger, J. (1964). Accidents des manipulations vertébrales. *J. Belg. Med. Phys.*

86 Pratt-Thomas, H.R. and Berger, K.E. (1947). Cerebellar and spinal injuries after chiropractic manipulation. *J. Am. Med. Assoc.*, **133**, 600

87 Pribek, R.A. (1962). Brainstem vascular accident following neck manipulation. *Wis. Med. J.*, **62**, 141

88 Richard, J. (1967). Disc rupture with cauda equine syndrome due to chiropractic adjustment. *NY State J. Med.*, **67**, 2496

89 Schwarz, G.A., Geiger, J.K. and Spano, A.V. (1956). Posterior inferior cerebellar artery syndrome of Wallenberg after chiropractic manipulation. *Arch. Intern. Med.*, **3**, 352

90 *Colt Symposium* (1982)

91 Maigne, R. (1968). *Douleurs d'origine vertebrale et traitement par manipulations.* (Paris: L'expansion)

92 Wyke, B.D. (1972). Articular neurology – a review. *Physiotherapy*, **58**, 94

93 Dee, R. (1969). Structure and function of hip-joint innervation. *Ann. R. Coll. Surg.*, **45**, 357

94 Roaf, R. (1978). *Posture*. (London: Academic Press)

95 Nicholls, P.J.R. (1960). Short-leg syndrome. *Br. Med. J.* June 18, 1863

96 Farfan, H.F. and Lamy, C. (1977). A mathematical model of the soft tissue mechanisms of the lumbar spine. In Buerger, A.A. and Tobis, J.S. (eds.) *Approaches to the Validation of Manipulation Therapy.* p. 5. (Springfield: Thomas)

97 Alexander, F.M. (1932). *The Use of Self.* (London: Methuen)

98 Barlow, E.D. and Pochin, E.E. (1948). Slow recovery from ischaemia in human nerves. *Clin. Sci.*, **6**, 303

99 Reading, A.E. (1977). Biofeedback training – an evaluation. *Hosp. Update*, **3**, 669

REFERENCES

100 Hurrell, M. (1980). Electromyographic feedback in rehabilitation. *Physiotherapy*, **66**, 293

101 Nathan, H. and Feuerstein, M. (1970) Angulated course of spinal nerve roots. *J. Neurosurg.*, **32**, 349

102 Brodal, A. (1965). *The Cranial Nerves – Anatomy and Anatomicoclinical Correlations.* (Oxford: Blackwell Scientific)

103 Brain, Lord and Wilkinson, M. (Eds.) (1967). *Cervical Spondylosis.* (London: Heinemann)

104 Andersson, B.J.G., Otengren, R. *et al.* (1974). On myoelectric back muscle activity and lumbar disc pressure in sitting postures. *Scand. J. Rehabil. Med. Suppl.*

105 Farhni, W.H. (1966). *Backache and Primal Posture.* (Vancouver: Musqueam Publishers)

106 McKenzie, R.A. (1977). Prophylaxis in recurrent low back pain. In *Proceedings: International Federation of Manual Medicine Congress, Copenhagen*

107 Nachemson, A. (1976). The lumbar spine; an orthopaedic challenge. *Spine*, **1**, 59

108 Weinstein, P.R., Ehni, G. and Wilson, C.B. (1977). Lumbar spondylosis: diagnosis, management and surgical treatment. (Chicago and London: Year Book Medical)

109 Hutton, W.C. and Adams, M.A. (1980). The forces acting on the neural arch and their relevance to low back pain. In *Conference Proceedings: Engineering Aspects of the Spine.* p. 49. (London: Mechanical Engineering Publications)

110 Wood, P.H.N. (1976). The epidemiology of back pain. In Jayson, M. (ed.) *The Lumbar Spine and Back Pain.* p. 13. (Tunbridge Wells: Pitman Medical)

111 Troup, J.D.G. (1979). Biomechanics of the vertebral column. *Physiotherapy*, **65**, 238

112 Davis, P.R. and Troup, J.D.G. (1966). Human thoracic diameters at rest and during activity. *J. Anat.*, **100**, 397

113 Newman, P.H. (1963). The aetiology of spondylolistheses. *J. Bone Jt. Surg.*, **45B**, 39

114 Hitselburger, W.E. and Witten, R.M. (1968). Abnormal myelograms in asymptomatic patients. *J. Neurosurg.*, **28**, 204

115 Porter, R.W., Wicks, M and Ottewell, D. (1978). Measurement of the spinal canal by diagnostic ultrasound. *J. Bone Jt. Surg.*, **60B**, 481

116 Vernon-Roberts, B. (1980). In Jayson, M. (ed.) *The Lumbar Spine and Back Pain.* 2nd Edn. (Tunbridge Wells: Pitman Medical)

117 Huskisson, E.C. (1974). Recent drugs and the rheumatic diseases. *Report on Rheumatic Disease No. 54.* (London: Arthritis and Rheumatism Council)

118 Dick, C.W. (1978). In Scott, J.T. (ed.) *Copeman's Textbook of the Rheumatic Diseases.* 5th Edn. (Edinburgh and London: Churchill Livingstone)

119 Lee, P. *et al.* (1974). Observations on drug prescribing in rheumatoid arthritis. *Br. Med. J.*, **1**, 424–6

120 Rooney, P.J. *et al.* (1975). A short term, double blind controlled trial of prenozone in rheumatoid arthritis. *Curr. Med. Res. Opin.* **2**, 43–50

121 Levy, M. *et al.* (1973). Aspirin use in patients with major upper gastrointestinal bleeding and peptic ulcer disease. *N. Engl. J. Med.*, **290**, 1158–62

122 Cameron, A.J. (1975). Aspirin & gastric ulcer. *Mayo Clin. Proc.* **50**, 565–70

123 Huskisson, E.C. and Grayson, M.F. (1974). Indomethacin or amylobarbitane sodium for sleep in rheumatoid arthritis with some observations on the use of sequential analysis. *Br. J. Clin. Pharmacol.*, **1**, 151–4

124 Hart, F.D. and Boardman, P.I. (1965). Indomethacin and Phenylbutazone – a comparison. *Br. Med. J.*, **2**, 1281–4

125 Jayson, M. (1982). Presentation at *Colt Symposium*

126 Calin, A. and Fries, J.F. (1975). Striking prevalence of ankylosing spondylitis in 'healthy' W27 positive males and females: a controlled study. *N. Engl. J. Med.*, **293**, 835

127 Wyke, B. (1965). Comparative analysis of proprioception in left and right arms. *Q. J. Exp. Psychology*, **17**, 149

128 Lee, C.K. and Lishman, R. (1975). Vision in movement and balance. *New Scientist*, **65**, 59

129 Perry, J. (1970). The use of external support in the treatment of low back pain. *J. Bone Jt. Surg.*, **52A**, 1440

130 Nachemson, A. and Lindh, M. (1969). Measurement of abdominal and back muscle strength with and without low back pain. *Scand. J. Rehabil. Med.*, **1**, 60

131 Walters, R.L. and Norris, J.M. (1970). The effects of spinal supports on the electrical activities of the trunk. *J. Bone Jt. Surg.*, **52A**, 51

132 Van Leuven, R.M. and Troup, J.D.G. (1969). The 'Instant' lumbar corset. *Physiotherapy*, **31**, 201

133 Norton, P.L. and Brown, T. (1957). The immobilising effect of back braces: their effect on the posture and motion of the lumbo-sacral spine. *J. Bone Jt. Surg.*, **39A**, 111

134 Nachemson, A. (1964). In vivo measurement of intra-discal pressure. *J. Bone Jt. Surg.*, **46A**, 1077

135 De Sèze, S. and Leverieux, J. (1951). Les tractions vertébrales; premières études expérimentales et résultats thérapeutiques d'après une expérience de quatre anées. *Sem. Hôp. (Paris)*, **27**, 2085

136 Nachemson, A. and Elfstrom, G. (1970). Intravital dynamic pressure measurements in lumbar discs. *Scand. J. Rehabil. Med.*, *Suppl.*, no 1

137 Mathews, J.A. (1968). Dynamic discography: a study of lumbar traction. *Ann. Phys. Med.*, **9**, 275

138 Weber, H. (1973). Traction therapy in sciatica due to disc prolapse. *J. Oslo City Hosp.*, **23**, 167

139 Keyserling, W.M., Herrin, G.D. and Chaffin, D.B. (1980). Isometric strength testing as a means of controlling medical incidents on strenuous jobs. *J. Occup. Med.*, **22**, 332–6

140 Nachemson, A.L. (1980). In Jayson, M. (ed.) *The Lumbar Spine and Back Pain.* 2nd Edn. (Tunbridge Wells: Pitman Medical)

141 Nachemson, A.L. (1976). In Jayson, M. (ed.) *The Lumbar Spine and Back Pain.* (Tunbridge Wells: Pitman Medical)

142 Lidstrom, A. and Zachrisson, M. (1970). Physical therapy on low back pain and sciatica. *Scand. J. Rehabil. Med.*, **2**, 37

143 Fordyce, W.E. *et al.* (1973). Operant conditioning in the treatment of chronic pain. *Arch. Phys. Med. Rehabil.*, **54**, 399

144 Mooney, V. and Cairns, D. (1978). Management in the patient with chronic low back pain. *Orthop. Clin. N. Am.*, **9**, 543

145 Mehta M. (1973). *Intractable Pain.* p. 147. (London: Saunders)

146 Black, R.G. and Bonica, J.J. (1973). Analgesic blocks. *Postgrad. Med.*, **53**, 105

147 Sunderland, S. (1978). Traumatised nerves, roots and ganglia; musculo-skeletal factors and neuropathological consequences. In Korr, I.M. (ed.) *The Neurobiologic Mechanisms in Manipulative Therapy.* p. 137. (London: Plenum)

148 Smythe, H.A. (1972). Non-articular rheumatism and the fibrositis syndrome. In Hollander, J.L. and McCarty, D.J. (eds.) *Arthritis and Allied Conditions*. 8th Edn. p. 874. (Philadelphia: Lea & Febiger)

149 Ingpen, M.L. and Burry, H.C. (1970). A lumbo-sacral strain syndrome. *Ann. Phys. Med.*, **10**, 270

150 Mooney, V.T. (1977). Facet pathology. In Kent, B. (ed.) *Proceedings: Third Seminar: International Federation of Orthopedic and Manipulative Therapists*. (Hayward, CA: IFOMT)

151 Gottesman, J.R., Harris, D.H. and Olshan, N.H. (1975). Suboccipital and cervical facet-joint injection complications. *Arch. Phys. Med. Rehabil.*, **56**, 539

152 Rees, W.S. (1971). Multiple bilateral subcutaneous rhizolysis of segmental nerves in the treatment of the intervertebral syndrome. *Ann. Gen. Pract.*, **16**, 126

153 Toakley, J.G. (1973). Subcutaneous lumbar rhizolysis – an assessment of 200 cases. *Med. J. Aust.*, **2**, 490

154 Burnell, A. (1974). Injection techniques in low back pain. In Twomey, L.T. (ed.) *Symposium: Low Back Pain*. p. 111 (Perth: Western Australia Institute of Technology)

155 King, J.S. (1977). Randomised trial of the Rees and Shealy methods for the treatment of low back pain. In Buerger, A.A. and Tobis, J.S. (eds.) *Approaches to the Validation of Manipulation Therapy*. p. 70. (Springfield: Thomas)

156 Oudenhoven, R.C. (1979). The role of laminectomy, facet rhizotomy, and epidural steroids. *Spine*, **4**, 145

157 Barbor, R. (1975). Presentation at *Reunión sobre Catalogia de la Columna Vertebral*, Murcia, March 1975

158 Hackett, G.S., (1958). *Ligament and Tendon Relaxation*. (Springfield: Thomas)

159 Melzack, R. (1975). The McGill pain questionnaire: major properties and scoring methods. *Pain*, **1**, 277

160 Bonica, J.J. (ed.) (1974). *International Symposium on Pain*. (New York: Raven Press).

161 Olivier, G. and Olivier, C. (1963). *Mécanique Articulaire*. Vol. 1, p. 185. (Paris: Vigot)

162 Kellgren, J.H. and Lawrence, J.S. (1958). Osteo-arthritis and disc degeneration in an urban population. *Ann. Rheum. Dis.*, **17**, 388

163 Fielding, J.W., Reddy, K. and Pappalardo, P. (1971). Fixed atlanto-axial rotatory subluxation. *J. Bone Jt. Surg.*, **53A**, 1031

164 Stillwell, D. (1956). Nerve supply of the vertebral column and its associated structures in the monkey. *Anat. Rec.*, **125**, 129

165 Wyke, B.D. (1979). Neurology of the cervical spinal joints. *Physiotherapy*, **65**, 72

166 Kimmel, D.L. (1961). Innervation of the spinal dura mater and dura mater of the posterior cranial fossa. *Neurology*, **11**, 800

167 Kottke, F.J. and Mundale, M.O. (1959). Range of mobility of the cervical spine. *Arch. Phys. Med.*, **40**, 379

168 Smith P., Benn R.T. and Sharp J., (1972). In *Copeman's Textbook of Rheumatic Diseases*, 5th Edn. (Edinburgh and London: Churchill Livingstone)

169 Keuter, E.J.W. (1970). Vascular origin of cranial sensory disturbances caused by pathology of the lower cervical spine. *Acta Neurochir.*, **23**, 229

170 Campbell, D.G. and Parsons, C.M. (1944). Referred head pain and its concomitants. *J. Nerv. Ment. Dis.*, **99**, 544

171 Trevor-Jones R, 1964. Osteo-arthritis of the paravertebral joints of the second

and third cervical vertebrae as a cause of occipital headaches. *S. Afr. Med. J.*, **38**, 392

172 Dutton, C.B. and Riley, L.H. (1969). Cervical migraine: not merely a pain in the neck. *Am. J. Med.*, **47**, 141

173 Magora, F. *et al.* (1974). An electromyographic investigation of the neck muscles in headache. *Electromyogr. Clin. Neurophysiol.*, **14**, 453

174 Friedman, A.P. (1975). Migraine. *Psychiatr. Ann.*, **5**, 29

175 Sheldon, K.W. (1967). Headache patterns and cervical nerve root compression – a 15-year study of hospitalisation for headache. *Headache*, Jan. 180

176 Cope, S. and Ryan, G.M.S. (1959). Cervical and otolith vertigo. *J. Laryngol. Otol.*, **73**, 113

177 Toglia, J.U., Rosenberg, P.E. and Ronis, M.L. (1969). Vestibular and audiological aspects of whiplash injury and head trauma. *J. Foren. Sci.*, **14**, 219

178 Kosoy, J. and Glassman, A.L. (1974). Audiovestibular findings with cervical spine trauma. *Tex. Med.*, **70**, 66

179 Dionne, J. (1974). Neck torsion nystagmus. *Can. J. Otolaryngol.*, **3**, 37

180 Jackson, R. (1967). Headaches associated with disorders of the cervical spine. *Headache*, **6**, 175

181 Roca, P.D. (1972). Ocular manifestations of whiplash injuries. *Ann. Ophthalmol.*, **4**, 63

182 Spisak, J. (1972). Bedeutung des segments C2–C3 im klinischen bild des akuten tortikollis. *Man. Med.*, **6**, 87

183 Gunn, C.C. and Milbrandt, W.E. (1976). Tennis elbow and the cervical spine. *Can. Med. Assoc. J.*, **114**, 803

184 Olsson, O. (1942). Arthrosis deformans des vorderen zahngelenkes. *Fortschr. Roentgen*, **66**, 233

185 Finneson, B.E. (1969). *Diagnosis and Management of Pain Syndromes*, 2nd Edn. (London: Saunders)

186 Phillips, D.G. (1975). Upper limb involvement in cervical spondylosis. *J. Neurol. Neurosurg. Psychiatry*, **38**, 386

187 von Torklus, D. and Gehle, W. (1972). *The Upper Cervical Spine* (London: Butterworth)

188 Swezey, R.L. and Silverman, T.R. (1971). Radiographic demonstration of induced vertebral facet displacement. *Arch. Phys. Med. Rehabil.*, **52**, 244

189 Sharp, J. and Purser, D.W. (1961). Spontaneous atlanto-axial dislocation in ankylosing spondylitis and rheumatoid arthritis. *Ann. Rheum. Dis.*, **20**, 47

190 Mathews, J.A. (1969). Atlanto-axial subluxation in rheumatoid arthritis. *Ann. Rheum. Dis.*, **28**, 260

191 Conlon, P.W., Isdale, I.C. and Rose, B.S. (1966). Rheumatoid arthritis of the cervical spine. *Ann. Rheum. Dis.*, **25**, 120

192 Whaley, K. and Dick, W.C. (1968). Fatal sub-axial dislocation of cervical spine in rheumatoid arthritis. *Br. Med. J*, **2**, 31

193 Wilkinson, M. (ed.) (1971). *Cervical Spondylosis: Its Early Diagnosis and Treatment*. 2nd Edn. (London: Heinemann)

194 Partridge, R.E. and Anderson, J.A. (1969). Back pain in industrial workers. *Proceedings of the International Rheumatology Congress*, Prague, Czechoslovakia, abstract 284

195 Magora, A. (1973). Investigation of the relation between low back pain and occupation. 4. Physical requirements: Bending, rotation, reaching and sudden maximal effort. *Scand. J. Rehabil. Med.*, **5**, 191–6

196 Braun, W. (1969). Ursachen des lumbalen Bandscheiberverfalls. In *Die Wirbelsäule in Forschung und Praxis*, p. 43

197 Svensson, H.-O. and Andersson, G.B.J. (1982). Low back pain in forty to forty-seven year old men. I. Frequency of occurrence and impact on medical services. *Scand. J. Rehabil. Med.* **14,** 47–53

198 Aaras, A. (1982). Presentation at *Colt Symposium*

199 Frykholm, R. (1951). Cervical nerve root compression resulting from disc degeneration and root sleeve fibrosis. *Acta Chir. Scand. Suppl.*, 160

200 Prinzmetal, M. and Massumi, R.A. (1955). The anterior chest wall syndrome: chest pain resembling pain of cardiac origin. *J. Am. Med. Assoc.*, **159,** 177

201 Allison, D.R. (1950). Pain in the chest wall simulating heart disease. *Br. Med. J.*, **1,** 332

202 Edwards, W.L.J. (1955). Musculo-skeletal chest pain following myocardial infarction. *Am. Heart J.*, **49,** 713

203 Fossgreen, J. (1984). Presentation at *BAMM Symposium*, London

204 Grant, A.P. and Keegan, D.A.J. (1968). Rib pain – a neglected diagnosis. *Ulster Med. J.*, **37,** 162

205 Marinacci, A.A. and Courville, C.B. (1962). Radicular syndromes simulating intra-abdominal surgical conditions. *Am. Surg.*, **28,** 59

206 Ashby, E.C. (1977). Abdominal pain of spinal origin. *Ann. R. Coll. Surg.*, **59,** 242

207 Nathan, H. *et al.* (1964). The costovertebral joints: anatomico-clinical observations in arthritis. *Arth. Rheum.*, **7,** 228

208 Nathan, H. and Schwartz, A. (1962). Inverted pattern of development of thoracic vertebral osteophytosis in situs inversus and in other instances of right descending aorta. *Radiol. Clin.*, **31,** 150

209 Scheuermann, H. (1921). Zur röentgensymptomatologie der juvelinen osteochondritis dorsi. *Z. Orthop. Chir.*, **41,** 305

210 Butler, R.W. (1955). The nature and significance of vertebral osteochondritis. *Proc. R. Soc. Med.*, **48,** 895

211 Stoddard, A. (1969). *A Manual of Osteopathic Practice.* (London: Hutchinson)

212 Scott, M.E. (1974). Spinal osteoporosis in the aged. *Aust. Fam. Phys.*, **3,** 281

213 Schmorl, G. and Junghans, H. (1956). *Clinique radiologie de la colonne vertébrale normale et pathologique: confrontation anatomico-pathologique.* p.137. (Paris: Doin)

214 Heylings, D.J.A. (1978). Supraspinous and interspinous ligaments of the human lumbar spine. *J. Anat.*, **125,** 127

215 Wyke, B.D. (1980). In Jayson, M.I.V. *The Lumbar Spine and Back Pain*, 2nd Edn. (Tunbridge Wells: Pitman Medical)

216 Epstein, B.S. (1969). *The Spine: a Radiological Text and Atlas.* 3rd Edn. (Philadelphia: Lea & Febiger)

217 La Rocca, H. and Macnab, I. (1969). Value of pre-employment radiographic assessment of the lumbar spine. *Can. Med. Assoc. J.*, **101,** 383

218 Kirkaldy-Willis, W.H. and Hill, R.J. (1979). A more precise diagnosis for low-back pain. *Spine*, **4,** 102

219 Weinstein, M.A. *et al.* (1975). Computed tomography in diastematomyelia. *Radiology*, **117,** 609

220 Horal, J. (1969). The clinical appearance of low back disorders in the city of Gothenburg, Sweden. *Acta Orthop. Scand. Suppl.*, 118

221 Magora, A. and Schwarz, A. (1976). Relation between the low back pain syndrome and X-ray findings. *Scand. J. Rehabil. Med.*, **8**, 115

222 Kettelkamp, D.B. and Wright, D.G. (1971). Spondylolisthesis in the Alaskan Eskimo. *J. Bone J. Surg.*, **53A**, 563

223 Sorenson, K.H. (1964) *Scheuermann's Juvenile Kyphosis.* (Munksgaard: Copenhagen)

224 Tilley, P. (1970). Is sacralization a significant factor in lumbar pain? *Colt Symposium*, **70**, 238–41

225 Dan, N.G. (1976). Entrapment syndrome. *Med. J. Aust*, **1**, 258

226 Shealy, C.N. (1974). Facets in back and sciatic pain. *Minn. Med.*, **57**, 199

227 Park, W.M. (1980). In Jayson, M.I.V. *The Lumbar Spine and Back Pain*, 2nd Edn. (Tunbridge Wells: Pitman Medical)

228 Yates, D.A.H. (1978). A comparison of the types of epidural injection commonly used in the treatment of low back pain and sciatica. *Rheum. Rehabil.*, **17**, 181

229 Yates, D.A.H. (1980). In Jayson, M.I.V. (ed.) *The Lumbar Spine and Back Pain.* 2nd Edn. (Tunbridge Wells: Pitman Medical)

230 Cyriax, J.H. (1975). *Textbook of Orthopaedic Medicine.* Vol. 1, 6th Edn. (London: Baillière Tindall)

231 Harley, C. (1966). Extradural corticosteroid infiltration. *Ann. Phys. Med.*, **9**, 22

232 Coomes, E.N. (1961). A comparison between epidural anaesthesia and bed rest in sciatica. *Br. Med. J.*, **1**, 20

233 Bradford, F.K. and Spurling, R.G. (1945). *The Intervertebral Disc.* 2nd Edn. (Springfield: Thomas)

234 Barr, J.S. (1951). Protruded discs and painful backs. *J. Bone Jt. Surg.*, **33B**, 3

235 Friberg, S. (1954). Lumbar disc degeneration in the problem of lumbago sciatica. *Bull. Hosp. Jt. Dis.*, **15**, 1

236 Rabinovitch, R. (1961). *Diseases of the Intervertebral Disc and its Surrounding Tissues.* (Springfield: Thomas)

237 Hirsch, C. (1965). Efficiency of surgery in low back disorders: pathoanatomical experimental and clinical studies. *J. Bone Jt. Surg.*, **47A**, 991

238 DePalma, A.F. and Rothman, R.H. (1970). *The Intervertebral Disc.* (Philadelphia: Saunders)

239 Solonen, K.A. (1957). The sacro-iliac joint in the light of anatomical roentgenological and clinical studies. *Acta Orthop. Scand. Suppl.*, 26

240 Weisl, H. (1955). The movements of the sacro-iliac joint. *Acta Anat.*, **23**, 80

241 Colachis, S.C., Warden, R.E. *et al.* (1963). Movement of the sacro-iliac joint in the adult male. *Arch. Phys. Med. Rehabil.*, **44**, 490

242 Frigerio, N.A., Stowe, R.R. and Howe, J.W. (1974). Movement of the sacro-iliac joint. *Clin. Orthop. Rel. Res.*, **100**, 370

243 Lewit, K. and Wolff, H.D. (1970). Conference on the pelvis. *Man. Med.*, **6**, 150

244 Mixter, W.H. and Barr, J.S. (1934). Rupture of intervertebral disc with involvement of the spinal cord. *N. Engl. J. Med.*, **211**, 210

245 Arnoldi, C.C. (1972). Intravertebral pressures in patients with lumbar pain: a preliminary communication. *Acta Orthop. Scand.*, **43**, 109

246 Kirkaldy-Willis, W.H. *et al.* (1974). Lumbar spinal stenosis. *Clin. Orthop.*, **99**, 30

247 Hudgins, W.R. (1977). The crossed straight-leg-raising test. *N. Engl. J. Med.*, **297**, 1127

248 Lansche, W.E. and Ford, L.T. (1960). Correlation of the myelogram with clinical and operative findings in lumbar disc lesions. *J. Bone Jt. Surg.*, **42A**, 193

249 Finneson, B.E. and Cooper, V.R. (1979). A lumbar disc surgery predictive score card: a retrospective evaluation. *Spine*, **4,** 141

250 Codman, E.A. (1934). *The Shoulder, Rupture of Supraspinatus Tendon and Other Lesions on or about the Sub-acromial Bursa.* (Boston, Mass.: Todd)

251 Mason, M. and Currey H.F.L. (eds.) (1976). *An Introduction to Clinical Rheumatology.* 2nd Edn. (Tunbridge Wells: Pitman Medical)

252 Cyriax, J.H. (1975). *Textbook of Orthopaedic Medicine.* Vol. 1, 6th Edn. (London: Baillière Tindall)

253 Thompson, T.C. and Doherty, J.H. (1962). Spontaneous rupture of the tendo achilles. A new clinical diagnosis test. *J. Trauma,* **2,** 126–9

254 Stamm, (1957). Surgical treatment of hallux valgus. *Group Hosp. Rep.,* **106,** 273

255 Cholmeley, (1955). Hallux valgus in adolescents. *Proc. R. Soc. Med.,* **51,** 905–6

256 Clarke, M. (1969). *Trouble with Feet.* (London: Bell)

Index